Treating Depression Naturally

*How Flower Essences Can Help
Rebalance Your Life*

Chris Phillips

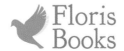

Floris
Books

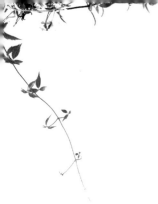

For Hedwig,
who helps my heart sing

First published in 2017 by Floris Books
© 2017 Chris Phillips

Chris Phillips has asserted his right under the
Copyright, Designs and Patent Act of 1988 to be
identified as the Author of this Work

 Also available as an eBook

British Library CIP data available
ISBN 978-178250-427-6
Printed in Great Britain
by Bell & Bain, Ltd

Note

Please note that the recommendations and case studies described in this book cannot replace the advice and treatment of a medical specialist. The author and publisher disclaim any warranty of fitness for a particular purpose and warn that readers should not rely on the content herein as a substitute for conventional medical treatment. For a correct diagnosis and appropriate treatment in the case of health problems, or suspected or existing illness, you should always seek the advice of your doctor/physician.

All reasonable efforts have been made to publish reliable data and information, but the author and publisher cannot assume responsibility for the validity of all materials or for the consequences of their use. The use of general descriptive names, trade names, trademarks, etc. does not imply that these names are protected by the relevant laws and regulations.

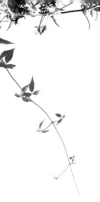

Contents

Part Three: The Road to Recovery

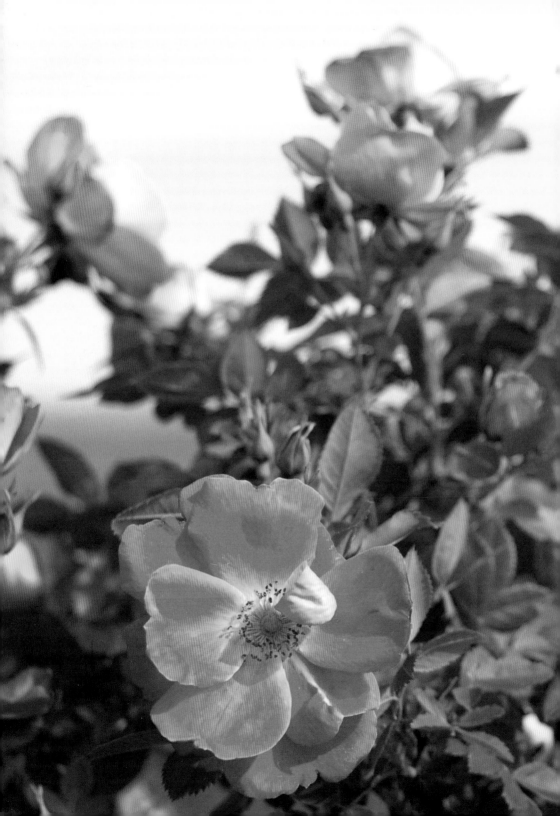

Foreword

How I came to flower essences

My wife Valerie was a very accomplished healer and for twenty years ran a busy private practice. In the winter of 1999/2000 she fell ill with cancer. To treat the pain, she surrounded herself with alternative therapists she felt comfortable with: a healer, a cranial osteopath and a reflexologist. Although she experienced many uncomfortable nights, she did not resort to morphine until the night before her death.

In the months that followed I suffered from the mixture of emotions that accompany mourning. My own health had been affected by my prolonged period as Valerie's nurse, but as I gradually recovered I wondered what further therapy might have helped Valerie, given her belief that conventional explanations about the onset of cancer left a lot unexplained. Her own healer had suggested she keep a journal during her illness and this included many recollections of her early life. Many of these were happy, but those stood out amongst other more challenging memories: of neglect by her mother and sexual abuse by her father, which I had known about but now seemed to be of even greater significance.

And then, almost two years to the day following Valerie's death, I came across a beautiful new book – *Bach Flower Remedies*[1] – about the healing properties of the Bach flowers. I read it as if it was the most gripping novel. Valerie and I had used the Bach remedies in the past and a therapy that enabled healing and growth across all levels of body, mind and spirit was exactly what I needed. I bought a box of the Bach remedies, and immediately started working on myself with them.

My first choice was **Wild Rose**, which Dr Bach wrote is for those who are:

> resigned to all that happens, and just glide through life, take it as it is, without any effort to improve things and find some joy. They have surrendered to the struggle of life without complaint.[2]

This describes a certain kind of depression that I had fallen into following Valerie's death. Gradually, on taking the remedy, I found myself coming back to life, and for the first time since she had died I experienced a sense of purpose. Other remedies followed – all had their part to play – but **Wild Rose** reset me on the right course and encouraged me to start advising relatives, friends and other people on how to use flower remedies.

I began to realise that I had a great deal more to learn from Dr Bach

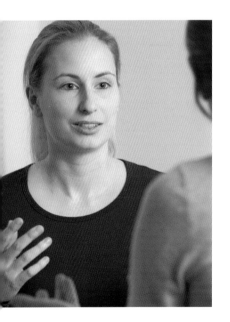

and his followers, much more than I had ever anticipated. I set out on my new career by adopting a mixture of practice (flower essences have no side effects – even a 'wrong' choice can have no ill outcomes, so my clients were safe at all times), reading, and courses and conferences. I also embraced psychotherapy, as that seemed directly relevant to what I was seeking to do.

It took me some years to discover that there was a professional organisation operating in the UK which supervised the standards of flower essence therapists: the British Flower and Vibrational Essence Association (BFVEA). By the time I came upon it I already had a useful amount of 'clinical' experience behind me, and I was able to make a case, in writing and by interview, which enabled me to become a practitioner member. The BFVEA acts as a forum for debate through regular meetings, and I find it extremely supportive.

What about conventional treatment?

In cases of significant illness it is always wise to visit your doctor. If depression or any other disorder is diagnosed, and medication recommended, there is nothing to stop you taking flower essences as well. Unlike some alternative treatments, flower essences do not conflict in any way with conventional medication.

In truth, flower essences bear only a tangential relationship to conventional medicine; their action is far wider. They are concerned with personal healing and growth at all levels of body, mind and spirit. And now, more than a dozen years since I started my new career, working a forty-hour week and having helped many hundreds of people, I feel truly blessed in my calling, and guided without cease by the flow of spirit within us all.

Flower essences can help to dampen the uncomfortable side effects of pharmaceutical drugs. Furthermore, pharmaceutical drugs frequently have significant withdrawal effects, so giving them up too early can be an uncomfortable and risky business. Despite feeling better, whether as a result of taking flower essences or not, it is always best to reduce your level of medication slowly and under supervision, and not before you have spent some weeks feeling ready to make the reduction.

Cognitive behavioural therapy and short-term counselling have also been shown to achieve results within a few sessions by modifying patients' behaviour, so these are the forms of psychotherapy the health profession most frequently turns to. Other forms of psychotherapy are seen to take longer and thus to cost more. My concern, and the concern of psychotherapists of all persuasions, is that depression is a problem of depth, and to go into depth takes time. When due time is taken, as happens in private-sector medicine, psychotherapy is frequently seen to work well. This is of course great if you can afford it – not everybody can. Here again, flower essence therapy has the ability to achieve maximum relief with minimum time and talking.

Chris Phillips, 2017

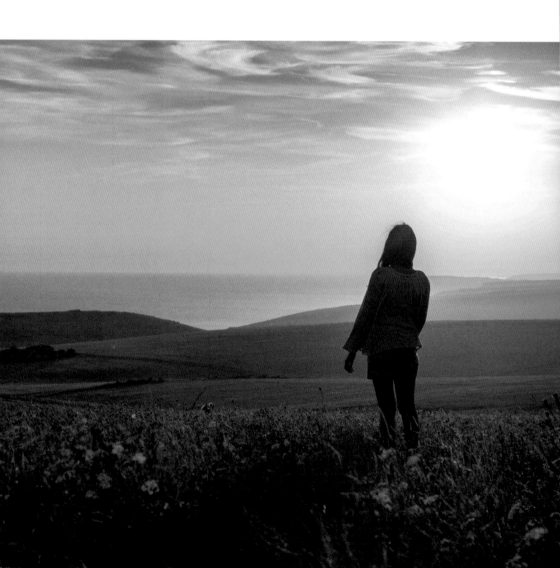

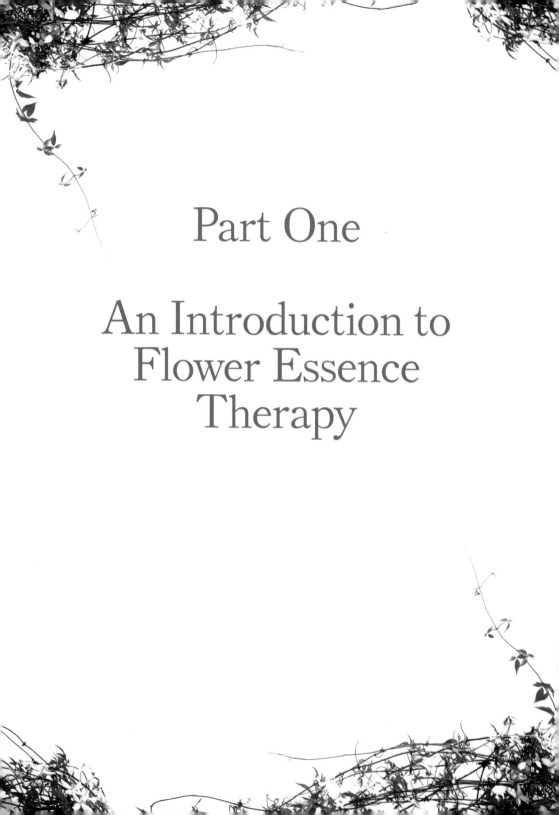

Part One

An Introduction to Flower Essence Therapy

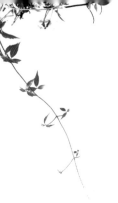

1
What is Depression?

There are 120 million people worldwide currently diagnosed with depression and it is estimated that in a few years it will become the world's most common chronic disease. But 'diagnosis' is a medical term – and there are many, many more cases of depression that are not diagnosed. The number of people who do not officially present with depression, and are therefore lost to the statistics, must be enormous.

Men get depressed too

While the majority of my clients are female, this may well be because men face much harsher stigma when speaking about their mental health, and therefore suffer in silence.

Before we begin, you may find it helpful to have some idea of how the medical profession categorises depression, which doctors and psychiatrists recognise is a unique experience, almost beyond classification.

Defining the undefineable

In typical mild, moderate, or severe depressive episodes, the patient suffers from lowering of mood, reduction of energy and decrease in activity. Capacity for enjoyment, interest and concentration is reduced, and marked tiredness after even minimum effort is common. Sleep is usually disturbed and appetite diminished. Self-esteem and self-confidence are almost always reduced and, even in the mild form, some ideas of guilt or worthlessness are often present. The lowered mood varies little from day to day, is unresponsive to circumstances and may be accompanied by so-called 'somatic' symptoms, such as loss of interest and pleasurable feelings, waking in the morning several hours before the usual time, depression worst in the morning, marked psychomotor retardation, agitation, loss of appetite, weight loss and loss of libido. Depending upon the number and severity of the symptoms, a depressive episode may be specified as mild, moderate or severe.[1]

The official definition above may well be helpful for the professionals, but I am assuming that you're reading this on the front line, as it were, struggling with the symptoms on a daily basis, and wanting to do something to fix the reason behind the depression rather than simply masking the symptoms. My belief is that we are here in this place, this universe, to discover and live up to the very best of our ability and potential, and when we are failing to do this we become unwell. Depression can be an indication that something is wrong in our lives.

A view of depression

Imagine aboriginal men and women forced to take shelter during the day in a dark cave, to escape a predator, bad weather, or an earthquake. Maybe they are hungry, cold and fearful, but at least they are safer than they would be outside, and their withdrawal from the light of day has given them a chance to regain their equilibrium.[2]

Dr David Rosen

Dr David Rosen, a Jungian analyst who I find constructive and sympathetic, is extremely positive about the opportunities inherent in depression, regarding, like Oscar Wilde, that 'where there is sorrow, there is holy ground'. He links depression to a way of adapting to different circumstances. This book uses Dr Rosen's approach, showing how we can work through our depression to regain that equilibrium and discover something new about ourselves.

Causes of depression

We don't get into depression without having prepared the ground beforehand, usually by sustaining some real difficulty in our early lives, difficulty so severe that it doesn't simply heal and go away. Studies have shown that infants and children who have been abused, neglected, lacked nurture, or experienced an emotional disturbance in some area of their lives are more likely to be depressed as adults. Nurture rather than nature seems to dominate in the development of depression.

The power of the brain

It is becoming increasingly clear that early nurture sets the thermostat for our levels of cortisol or patterns of brainwaves in the left frontal lobe. It is also becoming clear that subsequent good experiences, like therapy, can reset the levels to healthier ones.[3]

Oliver James

Importance of childhood

Children need security in order to thrive. Conflict and unkindness may be internalised by children and give rise to depression later on.

Being brought up in uncertainty or insecurity can inflict lifelong invisible but de-energising scars; as when, for example, there are unspoken conflicts in the parental relationship, or when one of the parents leaves the family several times. When they are very young, children's primary carers are essential to their physical and emotional survival, so to be unable to relate to them meaningfully has a powerful impact, which is hard to erase without significant help in future years. Oliver James also points out that 'being scripted to be a high achiever in the family drama' can also have a powerful effect on an individual.

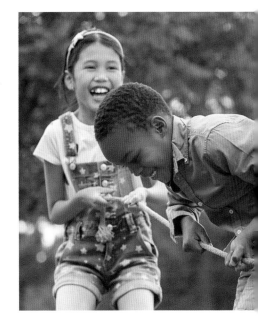

In later childhood, at a time when they should be learning about and exploring life's possibilities, some children are exposed to what they perceive as excessive constraint, usually from their parents. This can also be psychologically damaging. Excessive conflict between parents at this time can also send the message that relationships and love are hostile and even impossible.

The natural state of children is to be loving and generous, and they sometimes accept an amazing amount of unkind behaviour from their carers. But if the burden is too great it goes beyond their ability to process: they continue their psychological development *without* processing the damage they have sustained, and that damage can usually only be detected in bad behaviour, or perhaps not at all until years afterwards. The trauma acts as a blockage to their development, and remains unprocessed until later when some event occurs that acts as a trigger to the resulting depression. Often the event is either a loss of some kind, or is at least perceived by the person as a loss.

Of course, we should remember that no two children are alike. While one child may internalise an enduring trauma, another child in the same family may live through these same rugged conditions apparently without harm. All such difficulties can leave apparently indelible marks, distorting children's development, but also presenting valuable life challenges to be surmounted. These marks are not always easy to recognise or remove.

Therapy can help

Therapy can ease the burdens we acquire in childhood, dissolving the chains created by difficulties, and showing the way forward. Sensitive therapy can bring about a 'creation of home' for those who never had it.[4]

Alice Miller

While psychotherapy can be a long and sometimes expensive process, essence therapy is direct, gentle and affordable. The essences first dissolve, sometimes in days, psychic lesions that have lasted for years, and then patiently create and hold a space into which the person can grow.

Pre-birth trauma

In the womb, our unborn children are more aware of what is going on in the outer world than is usually imagined. If a mother experiences trauma – for example, losing her home or her partner unexpectedly, or the death of a loved one – this can affect the baby and lead to problems at the birth and later on. But I mention this pre-birth time particularly because there is one commonly recurring difficulty that has shown up a great deal in my work, particularly where depression occurs. I believe that when a baby is not wanted – either by its mother, father, or by close family members – the negative emotions this causes can sometimes be sensed by the unborn child. Children bring love into the world when they are born: the very idea of not being wanted is the antithesis of that love and is damaging to children's developing psyches.

It's not my intention, however, to blame mothers for this because many pregnant women find themselves in challenging situations outwith their control; this is simply part of life (see also Chapter 15).

Treatment

Even if antidepressants always did what they were supposed to do, and were always prescribed accurately (and depression is a particularly difficult ailment for a doctor or a psychiatrist to prescribe for precisely), there will always be a substantial shortfall between help needed and help received via the conventional medical route. Not to mention the fact that often these conventional treatments treat only the symptoms of depression and not the cause. However, natural treatments do exist and homeopaths and acupuncturists claim that they can alleviate many forms of depression.

Why try flower essences?

Flower essences are a therapy like no other where depression is concerned, because they work into the core of the problem.

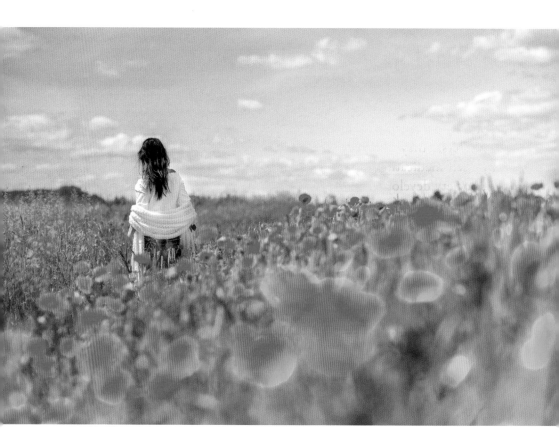

2

What are Flower Essences and How are they Used?

For thousands of years, when our distant ancestors lived as hunter-gatherers, they instinctively preserved or reclaimed their health by self-medicating on herbs and plants provided by nature. As society developed, so herbal medicine became our ancient pharmacy, usually composed of tinctures of the roots and stems and leaves and every part of a plant. Gradually, medical knowledge became the special preserve of particular individuals in tribes, villages or the cloister. We know that a few people had used the morning dew from flowers as healing elixirs: Hildegard of Bingen, a German healer, mystic and diviner working in the twelfth century and, four centuries later, Paracelsus, a renowned doctor from middle Europe. As these individual healers passed away, and the structure of society changed following the Industrial Revolution, during which many young people moved to cities, this ancient plant knowledge was often lost. Mainstream medicine and the pharmaceutical industry developed, and overshadowed ancient wisdom.

What is disease?

Disease will never be cured or eradicated by present materialistic methods, for the simple reason that disease in its origin is not material... disease is in essence the result of conflict between the soul and personality and will never be eradicated except by spiritual and mental effort.[1]

Dr Edward Bach

The person who is widely considered to have first (re)discovered and perfected flower essences for the Western world is Dr Edward Bach. Bach's work arose out of the tradition of homeopathy, which was developed more than two hundred years ago by Dr Samuel Hahnemann. Hahnemann had discovered the 'doctrine of similars', also known as 'like cures like'. In other words, medicines that provoked the symptoms of a particular disease would, when prescribed in small quantities, have a curative effect on that same disease.

Living longer

Bach believed very strongly that he averted his own death from cancer during this time by focusing all his energy during his 'last months of life' on the research he loved. He lived almost twenty years longer than predicted and made significant contributions to vaccine therapy and homeopathy during that time, as well as discovering flower remedies.

During the early 1900s, when still working in conventional medicine, Dr Bach made a significant contribution to vaccine therapy, and subsequently began preparing his material homeopathically. Nonetheless Bach felt that nature had something better in store. During a period of convalescence following illness, he had spent valuable time walking in the countryside and discovered some plants with interesting qualities, which he thought might bear further investigation. And so in 1930 he closed his lucrative London practice, and set out on a serious exploration.

Bach knew that he was looking for plants with a high healing potential, and as he searched he became more and more sensitive and intuitive, feeling the strong action of the plants he was drawn to. By the time of his death in 1936 his life's work was complete: his 38 remedies represented an entire new system of healing, and were available to the public at Nelson's homeopathic pharmacy in the West End of London.

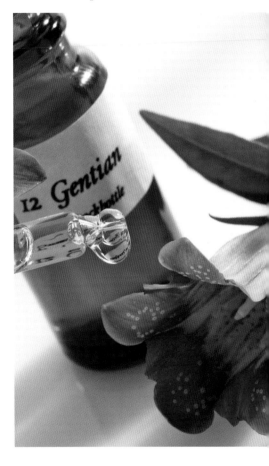

Matters remained more or less as they were for the next 31 years following Dr Bach's death. He had tried to bring the remedies to the attention of his colleagues without much success, and his advertisements to the public had incurred the wrath of the British Medical Association. However, in 1967 a different kind of doctor, a Yorkshireman with a PhD in electrical engineering, began to make new flower essences.

Arthur Bailey had discovered the Bach remedies during a particularly virulent and debilitating bout of Asian flu. He had been impressed, and started to prescribe the Bach remedies to others. Starting in his own garden, he gradually discovered other essences

23

which seemed to help his patients as well. Over time, a new range of essences was born: the Bailey Essences. Both Bach and Bailey essences are widely available and commonly used today.

How do flower essences work?

In the UK flower essences are officially classed as foods rather than medicines: they are harmless in all cases even if 'incorrectly' chosen, and recognised as being harmless by all governments. Nonetheless, there have been some encouraging organised studies into their worth. The British Association of Flower Essence Producers (BAFEP) carried out a survey using a methodology that concentrated on measuring people's subjective views of the effectiveness of the essences, which produced statistically significant, positive results. And the Flower Essence Society of California, the largest essence maker in the USA, sponsored five clinical studies a few years ago, specifically in the area of relieving depression, which again produced statistically significant, positive results.

Natural treatments can help

Even within the conventional medical community, there is a strong argument in favour of using natural treatments to help with depression.

An authoritative strand of the medical profession objects vigorously to the 'medicalisation' of depression – that process whereby complex mental health issues are seen purely as illnesses with biological causes treatable by drugs, rather than something that needs to be treated on a deeper level. There are therefore a number of reasons for adopting natural remedies as an antidote to depression.

It is true that severe depression stops you in your tracks, but one of the many charms of flower essences is that you can choose which to use.

As we shall see, they operate directly on energy, on moods such as low self-esteem or self-confidence, and on guilt and feelings of worthlessness. When you are entangled in these states sometimes – but by no means always – you can very clearly sense the negative emotion you are experiencing, and match this to the remedy you need to move through the symptoms of your depression, with complete safety.

Realigning your soul

I believe that, as with all species in nature, people share a common heritage that is defined for each one of us in a kind of blueprint, which we often call our soul. The soul does not only carry our spiritual self; it also holds this adaptable blueprint for each one of us, a representation of us in our perfection. And we humans have more options available to us than the other kingdoms of nature because we are creative: we can expand our consciousness and discover and promote change.

But as light floods in, shadows lengthen. Programmed to value change and expansion, we sometimes lose sight of our roots. In our struggle to achieve our potential, we tend to veer out of alignment with our soul purpose.

The longer we stay out of alignment the more we get used to it, and the more strongly we hang on to our misalignment. However, the universe (or God) has placed vibrational patterns in nature – patterns of stability and consistency that exist within all living beings and offer a healing potential that we can uncover, a way to realign ourselves. And it is these vibrational patterns which diligent flower essence makers have been unearthing for our benefit ever since the time of Dr Bach.

How flower essences are made

Take a thin glass bowl, fill with clear water from a stream or spring for preference, and float enough of the blooms of the plant to cover the surface. Allow this to stand in bright sunshine until the flowers begin to wilt. Very gently pick out the blooms, pour the water into bottles and add an equal quantity of brandy as a preservative. One drop alone of this is sufficient to make potent an eight-ounce bottle of water, from which doses may be taken by the teaspoonful as required.[2]

Dr Bach's instructions for making his remedies

Nowadays, thousands of flower essences are available and essence makers have experimented over the years: some make essences empowered by the light of the moon, which contributes a very different energy from those empowered by the sun. Others refuse to separate the flowers from the plant, and energise the water by pouring it over the blooms in situ, either in the wild or, for orchid essence makers, in the greenhouse. Another technique is to bend the flowers over into a bowl of water.

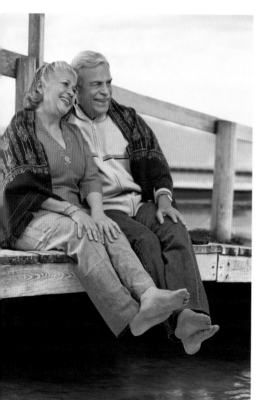

Water is the universal medium for holding the vibrational energy of the essence, but alcohol, whether brandy, vodka, or some other spirit, is almost universally added to keep the water clear of bacterial and fungal growth, and stabilise the energy (ch'i) of the flower.

There is a non-materialistic, numinous aspect to flower essence making. Patricia Kaminski of the Flower Essence Society of California writes that flowers should ideally be used just as they come to blossom, and with 'a deep seeing into the essence of the plant, a respect for and appreciation of its "creation song"'. We can draw the best medicine from plants when we commune and communicate with them in this ancient, almost religious way, 'where spirit and soul are not divorced from matter'.[3] Essence makers usually first research a plant's background and history before going into a reflective, meditative state to allow ideas about the plant's healing potential to come to them.

The medicine they produce, in turn, does not heal us directly, but acts as a catalyst for our soul's healing capacity, just like psychotherapy. In fact, they are used adjunctively in this way by many types of therapist.

Dealing with causes, not symptoms

Unlike conventional medicine, flower essences deal with causes rather than symptoms, depths rather than surfaces. I am not aware of another therapy that is so accessible and yet penetrates so quickly, directly and deeply to the source of our difficulties, and then dissolves them.

Selecting your essences

When I first started working with flower essences I hoped that a pattern in my work would emerge: first I would deal with this aspect, then with the next. But after a time I realised the pattern was a rather simple one: to deal with the immediate needs of the day. If you begin to detect movement in mood from day to day, this usually means movement towards better mental health. When this happens, you will begin to regain touch with various aspects of your personality, including painful aspects, which may have become dormant.

For example, an incident that you had not thought about for years, a real turning point in your life, may suddenly reappear in your consciousness, but without the attached emotional overload that it held then. You are able for the first time to see this important event from another perspective, allowing the remembered pain to dissolve. Perhaps you can even attribute value to what had been an awful event.

Focus on optimism

Look for a remedy to help with optimism rather than one that stops pessimism. Visualise, as clearly as you can, the type of emotional, physical, mental or spiritual relief you are looking for, then seek the essences to bring this change about.

Reducing stuckness

When being used to treat depression, as with any illness, the aim of flower essences is to reduce 'stuckness'. This is done by taking account of the most pressing feelings and applying essences to alleviate them. In due course, vital energy levels and the trust will lift.

A good way of reducing stuckness is to seek an essence simply to **improve your mood**. One that stops you feeling like a 'loser', or hopeless, or lonely, or however you may feel. Carl Jung talked about bringing his patients into a state of fluidity, where nothing is fixed. In a fluid state, change becomes possible.[4] The Bailey Essences recommend **Cyprus Rock Rose** for just this sort of thing:

Leave your fears behind

Cyprus Rock Rose (Bailey)
It is as if the flower says 'Stop – detach yourself from all your terrors and fears and spend a little time gathering together all you have learned in this life, all the wisdom and all the positive aspects of yourself.' In that insight you will discover that your hidden aspects are only fearful because they have been in the dark.[5]

Gradually, you will reach the point where you are no longer selecting essences to deal with the immediate, pressing difficulties of life, but creating greater happiness by choosing essences which support your **further development**, essentially your **creativity**. Bach's 'most creative' essence is **Wild Oat**. In its simplest interpretation, this remedy helps us to make choices about the work we do in life. Although, there are many, many essences that help in this important arena, because our work may well represent the utmost expression of our uniquely human spirit.

The universe wants to make itself known to those who can comprehend its language, and that language becomes more and more intelligible to us as our spiritual component unfolds.[6]

Itzhak Bentov in Stalking the Wild Pendulum

Next I suggest you consider whether **transition** essences are needed. Many essences can help guide us through the intense work necessary to process our pain, and among those I have found particularly helpful are:
- **Walking out of Patterns** (Dancing Light Orchid Essences)
- **Graceful Passages** (Star of California)
- **Walnut** (Bach)

When we experience significant developmental activity, even over many months, it can be valuable to take **stabilising** essences.

29

Change is not always easy and comfortable, and the safety and security of habit seeks to pull us back into old ways. I have found Perelandra's **Royal Highness** Rose helpful for stabilising the transformation experienced following a succession of essences.

Use your intuition

Dr Bach envisaged every home having a box of his remedies, which is why he provided brief and sensible booklets describing which symptoms each essence can be used for. But in fact, the essences can be used more widely than their descriptions suggest. Follow your intuition when selecting an essence, or you may be doing yourself a disservice. From reading a description of an essence you may simply feel a strong sense of this being the one for you. In which case, take it. If that feeling doesn't come, try to encourage a sense of openness as you browse. You may look at two or three essences or more and feel that any or all of them may be appropriate for you. It can help to sleep on your options, and in the morning you may find that you *know* which essence or essences you need. Of course, combining

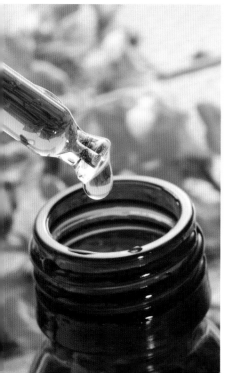

them all may be a perfectly valid response to your problem, though I'd advise you to limit it to six or seven at the most.

Flower essence practitioners commonly use intuition to select essences; they also use muscle testing, colour photo-cards of flowers (they seem to luminesce – or even repel – when you discover the essences you need), holding the patient's hand over a box of essences to see which essence feels right, and pendulum dowsing, which I personally use for remedy selection (see Resources). Not that you need to learn these techniques to choose useful essences for yourself; merely allowing yourself to 'feel' which essences are right for you at any particular moment can produce a rewarding outcome.

General relief

If the essences you apply from reading the chapters that follow do not seem to have the desired effect, turn to the following remedies and see if they offer any relief:

- **Formula Leucantha** (Florais de St Germain)
- **Red Helmet Orchid** (Australian Bush Flowers)
- **Splendid Mariposa Lily** (Flower Essence Services/FES)
- **Loved and Welcomed** (Flower Essences of Fox Mountain)

How to use remedies

Once you have decided which essence or essences you would like to work with, use the Resources chapter to source them. When you have them to hand, put a few drops, say seven, of each into a glass with very little water, and drink it. Do this twice a day: first thing in the morning and last thing at night. If you prefer to take fewer drops, or to take the essences more frequently, then do so.

Regularity is more important than frequency.

If you feel significantly better after a while, don't stop, but continue taking the essences. Usually a period of around three weeks is sufficient to consolidate the changes you are seeking to bring about, but, again, allow yourself to be influenced by your own feelings and instincts.

Recommended essence makers

Bach Remedies

The original flower essences discovered by Dr Bach, now made by Nelsons as well as a number of other producers. My preferred maker is Julian Barnard of Healing*herbs*, located in Herefordshire. **www.healingherbs.co.uk**

Bailey Essences

Developed by Arthur Bailey from 1967 until just before his death in 2007. The company is now run by his widow, Chris, and essence maker Jenny Howarth. Bailey Essences link with traditional Chinese medicine (TCM) by providing a 'five-element' set of essences. **www.yorkshirefloweressences.com**

Australian Bush Flowers (Bush)

Developed by the naturopath and herbalist Ian White, who travels the world indefatigably, giving courses and spreading knowledge about his essences. He has written a number of detailed and useful books on the Australian Bush Flowers.
www.universalessences.com (UK distributor)
www.ausflowers.com.au (Australian)

Flower Essences Services (FES)

This range has been developed over many years by Richard Katz and Patricia Kaminski of California, who have become the largest North American essence maker. They have a large range of their own and market Healing*herbs* throughout their region, as well as teaching and writing extensively.
www.universalessences.com (UK distributor)
www.fesflowers.com (International)

Pacific Essences

Located on Vancouver Island, these are made by Sabina Pettitt, who has dovetailed her flower and sea essence making into her work as an acupuncturist over many years.
www.essencesforlife.co.uk (UK distributor)
www.pacificessences.com (International)

I also include some particular favourite essences from other makers, which have emerged over the years as especially useful in treating varieties of depressive illness. I have made further recommendations for useful websites at the back of the book (see p. 208). But these are only my choices; there are many others out there – too many for me to include them all – and they also produce excellent essences.

If an essence comes your way and you feel inclined to try it, don't avoid it because it doesn't appear in this book. Follow your own intuition wherever possible; take it and see what happens. You can be sure it won't harm you, and it may do you a great deal of good.

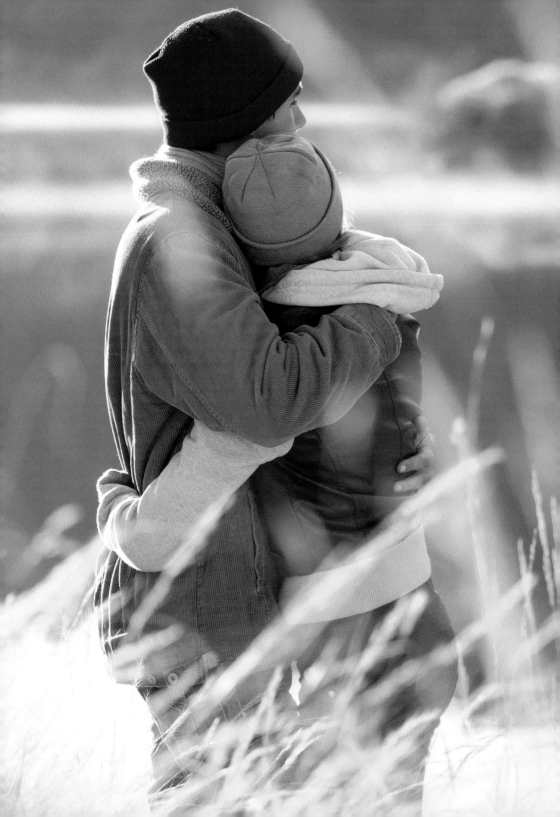

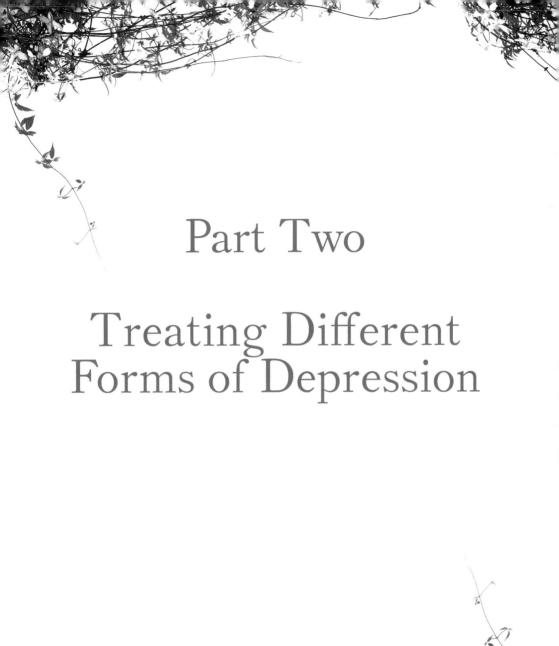

Part Two

Treating Different
Forms of Depression

How to Use Part Two

Until this point I have written about depression as if it were a single disorder, but of course it is not. The umbrella term 'depression' can be used to describe a huge range of mental disorders. In truth we should not even be confining ourselves to discussing mental disorder: depression afflicts us in so many physical ways that the diagnosis of depression is a constant challenge to even the most gifted doctor or psychiatrist. But for the sake of practicality and usefulness I have divided up the various symptoms and manifestations that tend to accompany depression, so that you can read about the symptoms you are experiencing and find the most suitable flower essences.

I have omitted some more severe mental illnesses, such as schizophrenia, bi-polar disorder and psychosis – not because flower essences are unable to help with these conditions, but because they are complex and would be best treated by a doctor and a flower essence practitioner, rather than through the pages of a reference book.

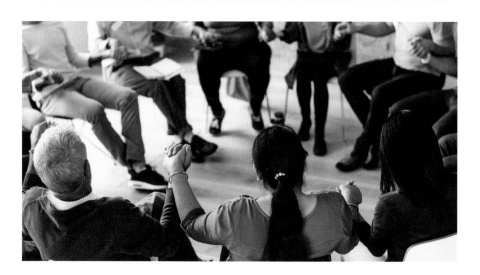

3
General Depression and Anxiety

Depression can seem difficult to categorise and almost impossible to describe. My own experiences of depression have also varied hugely, so each individual's experience must vary even more so from another's.

Experiencing depression

> Severe depression is a weird state – if you can describe your depression you almost certainly have not truly experienced it... It deserves some new and special word of its own, a word that somehow encapsulates both the pain and the conviction that no remedy will ever come.[1]

Lewis Wolpert

At the age of seventeen I sat in my room feeling the utter pointlessness of life, such a sense of paralysing despair that I was unable to move from my chair. I now know very clearly that I was undergoing a brief but intense depressive episode. But this was nothing like my experience 25 years later.

I was dragging myself into my office as if I was weighed down by a great and invisible burden. I functioned, bowed down at my desk and worked excessively slowly, breaking each task in front of me into the tiniest components. I would locate a telephone number, lift the handset, key the numbers – each action at the limit of my ability – and then have a perfectly sensible conversation, seemingly vitalised by the other person's energy.

These two experiences were very different. In the second I did not feel the worthlessness of living that characterised the first, and yet they were both instances of depression experienced by the same individual. Likewise, the resolution of each episode was utterly different. In the first I recall that although I had been feeling low for some time beforehand, I only plumbed the depths on that one afternoon. As I sat there in desperation I was, really quite suddenly, visited by a blessed sense of relief, a conviction of absolute certainty that life was all right and worthwhile and there to be lived. It seemed that almost within minutes my spirits were restored. Reflecting upon the experience afterwards I felt that I had been touched by God's grace. Not so with the later experience. It took me some months to gradually recover and function fully in a normal manner. I wish I had known then what I know now about flower essences – the whole process could have been resolved with much less pain and difficulty.

Recognising anxiety

Anxiety is a more visible ailment than depression; perhaps easier to recognise and diagnose, but capable of being just as debilitating. My clients report their anxiety to me much more frequently than their depression, yet anxiety is often present within depression.

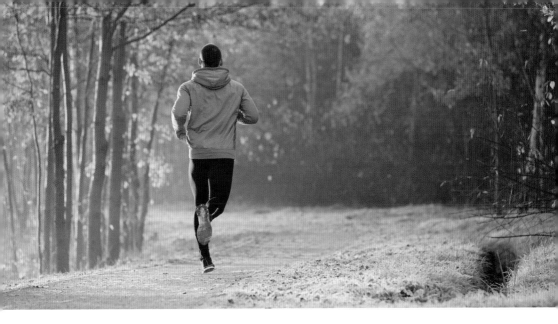

Of itself, anxiety is not an unhealthy state. The symptoms of anxiety are remarkably like those of **fear**, which is a normal response to threatening situations, and keeps us alert and prepared to deal with danger. But when it is so frequent and persistent that it interferes with normal activities, it's time to seek help. In its severest form, a feeling of dread can take over. My dictionary summarises dread as 'a state of chronic apprehension as a symptom of mental disorder'.

Symptoms of anxiety

As with depression, symptoms are not reliably consistent, but include feelings of:

- panic, fear and unease
- problems sleeping
- cold or sweaty hands or feet
- heart palpitations
- a dry mouth
- numbness
- tingling in hands or feet
- nausea
- muscle tension
- dizziness
- incontinence

If anxiety is so similar to fear, it's worth asking the following questions:

- What is the person afraid of?
- Where does the fear originate?
- Why does the same experience evoke fear in one person but not another?

The scientific jury is still out on these questions, but it does seem clear that anxiety lies in the individual's perception. And we do know that the roots of our anxiety go back a long way, perhaps to childhood, or even earlier.

For whatever reason, some children feel they can only rely on themselves. Even if their situation improves, the seed is sown in early life that they must do everything alone. Later on, when they find themselves unable to control every element of life, as of course no one can, they feel frightened, and anxious, and panic.

Case study: Diana
Anxiety hiding behind cheerfulness

Some people mask their anxiety very well. They appear to be very happy on the surface. When Diana first saw me her vital energy level was very low. Her fears were manifested in a terror of the dentist. Her pattern was to overwork to exhaustion, at which point she suffered pain and headaches, but she always maintained a smiling face to the world and calmly carried on with her day job. Despite her very low vital energy, she had recently discovered her unusual and fulfilling life purpose and, in her free time, was working at it as hard as she could.

She went on to tell me that her elder twin had died at birth, which was the probable cause of her later difficulties. She had been anorexic, suffered **panic attacks** – another form of extreme anxiety – and felt suicidal after her marriage breakdown. She had sustained a number of accidents and been temporarily paralysed following one of them. She had also become addicted to tranquillisers, and she had self-harmed in the past.

This particular form of anxiety – panic attacks, as well as **specific fear** – is a very close fit to Bach's **Agrimony** remedy, which is for 'anxiety, hidden by a mask of cheerfulness'. His description matches Diana almost perfectly:

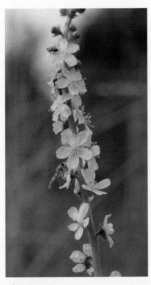

The **Agrimony** personality appears happy, enthusiastic, popular and seemingly at peace with the world. However, if one is able to know such a person on a deeper level, it becomes clear that something is deeply troubling the soul. At the heart of such suffering is a secret torment that is hidden, not only from others, but most importantly from the Self. There may be a strong attraction to drugs ... in order to maintain the mask of cheerfulness.[2]

Agrimony

I think that, for Diana, the 'secret torment that was hidden from her Self' was the traumatic early death of her twin: I believe it invisibly coloured the rest of her life. Her seemingly cheerful nature concealed this for a long time, and **Agrimony** would encourage the steadfast peace for which she secretly longed.

I gave her **Agrimony**, supported by **Olive** for **exhaustion**, and also **Willow**, which as Dr Bach put it, is for those who 'feel that they have not deserved so great a trial, that it was unjust, and they become embittered'. By her second session she was feeling a lot better, but her fear of the dentist had become the big issue. I added the Alaskan flower essence, **False Hellebore**, which 'promotes the release of false concepts; catalyses movement from the old to the new; helps us face our deepest, darkest fears'. She told me later that she eventually faced the dentist with complete confidence, and by this point her energy level was very good.

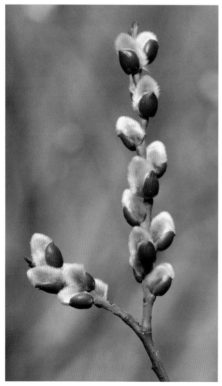

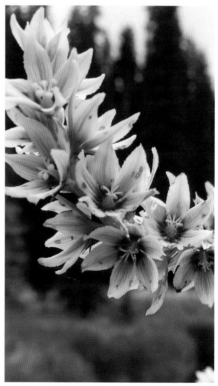

Willow

False Hellebore

Case study: Gina
Severe depression and anxiety

Gina came to see me when she was experiencing **severe depression** and **anxiety**. She had been unemployed for some time, and was taking sleeping tablets and an antidepressant. Her energy level was very low.

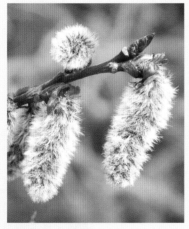

Aspen

Her anxiety was non-specific, and at her most stressed point she had suffered a debilitating breakdown. Bach's **Aspen**, a remedy for **inexplicable fear and dread**, seemed the most applicable to her condition. Writer and essence maker Julian Barnard says Bach wrote of 'vague unexplainable fears' that 'may haunt by night or day ... and have no rational explanation'.[3]

I also gave Gina **Cherry Plum**, which addresses the fear of doing dreaded things and brings us back to calmness and sanity. People in the negative **Cherry Plum** state lose all connection with the guidance of their Higher Self, and therefore of their destiny.[4] When Gina had a breakdown previously,

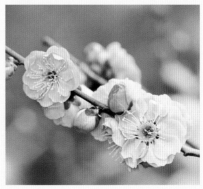

Cherry Plum

before I first met her, it had been sudden, irrational and terrifying, and there had been no guarantee of it not being repeated. **Cherry Plum** remedies this state. Complementing this, I gave Gina:

- **Gentian** (Bach) to help build perseverance
- **Gorse** (Bach) for hopelessness, for the feeling that there is no point in trying. Dr Bach listed it as one of his 'seven helpers', remedies that addressed chronic, long-standing conditions.

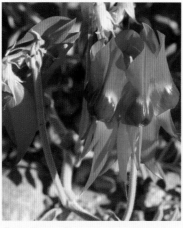

Sturt Desert Pea

A few weeks later Gina was suffering from bronchitis, for which I gave her **Sturt Desert Pea** 'for deep hurts and sorrows'. Two things from Gina's past had come to the surface: the first, that Gina's mother had been initially unhappy about motherhood; and the second, that Gina herself had never properly mourned the break-up of her marriage. In traditional Chinese medicine (TCM) **grief** is associated with the lungs, and I believe the bronchitis appeared to signal it was time for her severe and long-standing grieving to be resolved. When I saw her a year later, I found that Gina's health had improved so much that she had stopped taking any medication and taken on a demanding new job.

Treatment

From reading these case studies, and from my own experience, it is clear that the terms 'general depression' and 'anxiety' cover a broad range of complex mental states. Fear, which is a great antagonist to love, often emerges as the culprit, successfully steering victims away from their true path in life or hampering them from achieving fulfilment. Ian White, maker of the Australian Bush Flower essences, writes that fear has the effect of blocking and suppressing the life force, the vital energy.[5] The following table lists the essences I would suggest you consider for general depression, anxiety, dread and worry, to open you up to higher energies:

The descriptions of symptoms are brief, but hopefully one or more will resonate with you, and the essences may prove useful.

Feel free to experiment!

The technique of matching essences to mental and emotional conditions is called 'repertorising' and some essence therapists feel it is limiting because the essences are wonderfully flexible and work uniquely for each person who takes them, so think 'outside the box'.

It is also worth noting that some makers produce composite remedies, made up from several essences. Bailey Essences, for example, offers **Depression and Despair**, which includes the individual essences **Blackthorn**, **Bluebell**, **Hawkweed** and **Flowering Currant**. And they have a **Fears** composite, which includes **Betony**, **Greater Celandine** and **Mahonia**.

Turn to page 202 to find out more about selecting and sourcing these essences.

Symptoms	Remedy
Worry hidden by a carefree mask, apparently jovial but suffering	**Agrimony** (Bach) for steadfast peace
Vague, haunting apprehension and premonitions	**Aspen** (Bach) for trusting the unknown

Symptoms	Remedy
Fear of losing control, doing dreaded things	**Cherry Plum** (Bach) for steadfast peace
Discouragement, despondency, doubt	**Gentian** (Bach) for taking heart and having faith
Hopelessness, pointless to try	**Gorse** (Bach) for renewing
Fear of specific, known things; animals, heights, pain etc.	**Mimulus** (Bach) for bravery
Sudden gloom for no apparent reason	**Mustard** (Bach) for clarity
Feeling alarmed, intensely scared, horror, dread	**Rock Rose** (Bach) for the courage to face an emergency
Needing physical and mental renewal	**Olive** (Bach) for rest and support
Dissatisfied, bitter, resentful	**Willow** (Bach) for uncomplaining acceptance
Deep, unrecognisable fears	**Betony** (Bailey) for the glory of being alive
The deepest depths of despair	**Blackthorn** (Bailey) for transition to a new way of living
Deep terrors and fears that are difficult to expose and resolve	**Cyprus Rock Rose** (Bailey) for breakthrough and total transformation
Complete loss of heart, feeling of facing inevitable defeat	**Flowering Currant** (Bailey) for letting go of fears
Constant worry, a wandering mind	**Hairy Sedge** (Bailey) for anchoring the mind in the present
Times of major upheaval when we feel disoriented and lost	**Rosebay Willowherb** (Bailey) for going out into the world with confidence
Continual worrying	**Crowea** (Bush) for being balanced and centred
Fear of losing control	**Dog Rose of the Wild Forces** (Bush) for being calm and centred
Little desire to move	**Flannel Flower** (Bush) for joy in physical activity

Symptoms	Remedy
Despondency, gloom and resignation	**Kapok Bush** (Bush) for willingness and persistence
Disheartened, sluggish and weary	**Old Man Banksia** (Bush) for renewed enthusiasm
Deep hurt going back a long time	**Sturt Desert Pea** (Bush) for releasing deep-held grief and sadness
Loneliness and alienation	**Tall Yellow Top** (Bush) for a sense of belonging
Despair	**Waratah** (Bush) for courage, tenacity and adaptability
Depressed by the ugliness of urban culture	**Desert Lily** (FES) for the ability to radiate beauty within the mechanised urban environment
Intellect develops faster than emotions, ADHD tendency	**Downy Avens** (FES) for intelligence integrated with head and heart
Chronic anxiety and worry	**Garlic** (FES) for vital response to life
Deep depression	**Milkweed** (FES) for compassionate acceptance of life
Feeling of personal devastation	**Sagebrush** (FES) for the capability to transform
Discouragement in the face of obstacles	**Scotch Broom** (FES) for optimism about the future
Lack of vitality in speaking	**Trumpet Vine** (FES) for dynamic projection of oneself
Constraint, fear of being noticed	**Bluebell** (Pacific) for the ability to express our uniqueness
Mental darkness and despair	**Fairy Bell** (Pacific) for light-hearted release; willingness to follow your guidance
Dark cloud of depression	**Periwinkle** (Pacific) for finding our own deepest wisdom

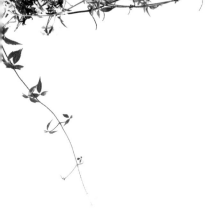

4
Chemically Induced Depression

The chemical inducement I'm referring to here is usually pharmaceutical or recreational drugs, or alcohol. Addiction to stimulants seems to deplete love and increase fear, making the world a bleaker place.[1] Joy departs and darkness moves in, cynicism abounds and trust is lost. This is why the 'twelve steps' programmes of Alcoholics and Narcotics Anonymous have such an overtly spiritual message. For example, Step 11 states that we have 'sought through prayer and meditation to improve our conscious contact with God as we understood Him'. It is one thing to give up drugs or alcohol, but the aching void maintained or created by the addiction also needs to be dealt with, and spiritual faith has the depth to fill the void.

Case study: Brenda
Feelings of worthlessness, alcoholism

I first saw Brenda when she had been diagnosed with cervical cancer and was facing an intensive programme of **chemo and radiotherapy**. She was a recovering **alcoholic** and had worked through Alcoholics Anonymous. She had suffered for as long as she could remember from a feeling of **worthlessness**, and confessed to feeling terrified at her current situation. I gave her **Tomato** and **Date** from Spirit in Nature essences. **Tomato**

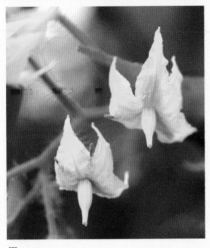

acts on all levels of fear and weakness, and on addiction and defensiveness. Its outcomes are mental strength, courage and belief in oneself. **Date** helps those who are judgemental and critical of others to be more tender and forgiving; it helps too with self-nurture.

This remedy was too strong for Brenda, however, and she couldn't sleep after taking it. Even reducing the

Tomato

dose to one drop was too much. Her resistance was simply too strong, and we did not work together again for a year.

However, she did come back and when I next saw her she was still suffering from a feeling of unworthiness, but her main complaints were:

- 🌸 weariness, for which I gave her **Hornbeam** (Bach)
- 🌸 no love or joy in living – **Wild Rose** (Bach)
- 🌸 unendurable desolation – **Sweet Chestnut** (Bach)

This steadied her during the next few weeks and her energy improved, though her sense of unworthiness persisted. Her next batch of remedies came from the Pacific Essences range:

- 🌸 **Poison Hemlock** for transition and letting go
- 🌸 **Nootka Rose** for love of life, laughter and joy following major trauma (in this case from her youth)

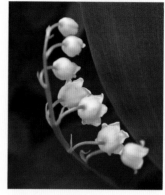

🌸 **Lily of the Valley**, which 'brings us back to that state of child-like innocence and wisdom where we only know how to respond with loving behaviour'

Again her energy improved, as did her trust in life, and we finally managed to tackle her persistent sense of unworthiness.

Lily of the Valley

Treatment

Reducing fear, supporting love, and dissolving addiction and trauma are the main issues to address. Many of the essences listed in Chapter 3 will also be suitable for chemically induced depression, so do look at them as well. Turn to page 202 to find out more about selecting and sourcing these essences.

Symptoms	Remedy
Jealousy, envy, revenge, anger and suspicion	**Holly** (Bach) for conquering it all through love
Weary, unable to cope	**Hornbeam** (Bach) for strength and support
Expecting to fail, lacking confidence and the will to succeed	**Larch** (Bach) for self-confidence, willingness to try anything
Unendurable desolation	**Sweet Chestnut** (Bach) for a light shining in the darkness
Not interested in life, resignation, no point in life	**Wild Rose** (Bach) a spirit of joy and adventure

Symptoms	Remedy
Deep terrors and fears that are difficult to expose and resolve	**Cyprus Rock Rose** (Bailey) for breakthrough and total transformation
Addiction is a family pattern	**Boab** (Bush) for breaking free from addiction
Sabotage of self or goals	**Five Corners** (Bush) for building up self-esteem
Vague, disconnected (over 28 years old)	**Red Lily** (Bush) for grounding after drug use
Vague, disconnected (under 28 years old)	**Sundew** (Bush) for focus, attention to detail
Crisis due to overly materialistic focus	**Chrysanthemum** (FES) for transcendent soul expression
Dependence on drugs for protection or social masking	**Golden Yarrow** (FES) for being open to others while staying self-contained
Lack of joy, warmth and vitality in sexual expression	**Hibiscus** (FES) for warmth and responsiveness in sexuality
Sexual behaviour divorced from human love	**Sticky Monkeyflower** (FES) for expressing love in sexual relationships
Fear due to overly materialistic focus	**Trillium** (FES) for sense of financial well-being
Endless mental darkness	**Fairy Bell** (Pacific) for finding the light
Stuck within your Self	**Harvest Lily** (Pacific) for finding a sense of community
Over-control, rigidity	**Lily of the Valley** (Pacific) for simplicity, innocence, unconditional love
Abuse, abandonment; psychological, emotional or physical assault	**Nootka Rose** (Pacific) for expressing love of life, laughter and joy
Major trauma	**Poison Hemlock** (Pacific) for transition and letting go
Energy blockages, restrictive personal patterns	**Snowdrop** (Pacific) for letting go, having fun, lightening up

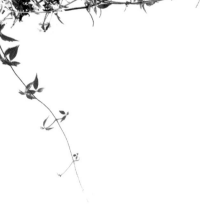

5
Obsessive Compulsive Disorder (OCD)

OCD seems to arise as a pathological attempt at controlling our environment. That desire to control, apparently beyond all reason, appears to come from a deep childhood need to manage the world around us. It's hard to pinpoint exactly what causes OCD, and several different factors may play a role. One of these is trauma in early childhood, for example, arising from bullying, neglect, abuse or bereavement. When early childhood trauma of this nature is experienced – in which we feel that if we don't control events then no one else will – the urge to seize control can develop very early on.

Find your inner strength

The 'antidote' is therefore to discover that love and support are inherent within us and in the universe around us. Flower essences can help us to uncover our inner strength.

This is why small but compelling and all-consuming OCD rituals often seem so bizarre: they appear to be impulses from long ago when we were very small. At the time, the originating trauma was promptly buried in our subconscious and forgotten, as we all do so very well. But trauma, unobserved, lives on, guiding our development in unexpected ways. People diagnosed with OCD (as well as autism) often develop a special affinity for work in the fields of computing and robotics, and put their supposed deficiencies to good use. But sometimes the affliction is too great, and people can feel effectively locked out of the world.

Case study: Terry
OCD, extreme anxiety

Terry was referred to me suffering from **extreme anxiety**, and had been diagnosed as being high on the autistic spectrum. His IQ seemed to be normal for his age (he was seventeen at the time) and he was receiving no medication. He became very agitated if he had to leave the house without first going sequentially through an elaborate ritual. In addition to this, between the ages of seven and fourteen he had felt constrained by his parents in his daily life. None of this necessarily reflects abusive parenting: he may quite simply have been hard to handle at home. But, nonetheless, this **parental constraint** rankled and he had internalised it in a way that reinforced his anxiety, which mainly manifested in the form of OCD.

The remedy I gave him first was Arthur Bailey's **grief**-specific essence, **Yorkshire Fog**, which enables us to open up to the pain of grief and to shed tears that wash away our anger, frustration and sadness.[1] When as children we fall and bruise ourselves, we cry, we seek help, we are comforted, we run off and continue with the game and the bruise quickly heals. But if an inner hurt occurs, which for some reason we cannot acknowledge, that inner bruise may not heal at all, sometimes for a lifetime, and our energy remains depleted by the internal wound. This remedy seemed to serve Terry well. I followed it up some weeks later with **Purple Monkeyflower** from the Flower Essence Society, which addresses a state of fear within the soul by **engendering courage** in the recipient who can then 'find true spiritual guidance, sustenance and support for life on Earth'.[2] Soon afterwards

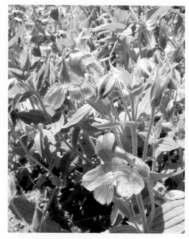

Purple Monkeyflower

Terry was no longer feeling anxious and, interestingly, he was also dealing better with his autism.

Treatment

The following table goes on to list a range of symptoms that those with OCD may suffer. From my experience, difficulties internalised during childhood often lie buried at the root of illnesses such as OCD.

Since I met with Terry, a new remedy has been produced by Florais de St Germain called **Formula Leucantha**, which is made up of a number of Brazilian flowers that work together to allay a paralysing **sense of loss**. Frequently, I use **Red Helmet Orchid** (Bush) to complement **Formula Leucantha**, as this orchid deals very specifically with **father issues**.

Although childhood trauma often lies buried, a sense of alienation may remain as a clue, some feeling of loss that you have been unable to put your finger on.

Are you suffering from all-consuming OCD?

If OCD is quite literally preventing you from getting on with your life, and if you have any suspicion at all of early childhood loss, try **Formula Leucantha** and the **Red Helmet Orchid**.

No harm will come to you if these remedies are not needed, but if they are, you may experience a real benefit and a consequent lift in energy. You can also use your intuition to choose from the following suggestions. Turn to page 202 to find out more about selecting and sourcing these essences.

Symptoms	Remedy
Obsession with impurities, diet, hygiene or personal faults	**Crab Apple** (Bach) for mental, emotional and physical cleansing
Extreme fear	**Rock Rose** (Bach) for the courage to face any emergency
Constraint, self-denial, rigidity	**Rock Water** (Bach) for broadening outlook, understanding
Repetitive, circling thoughts	**White Chestnut** (Bach) for a calm, clear mind
Deep terrors and fears that are difficult to expose or resolve	**Cyprus Rock Rose** (Bailey) for breakthrough and total transformation
Anger, frustration and sadness of grief	**Yorkshire Fog** (Bailey) for expressing grief, not being entangled by it
Obsessive infatuation and repetitive thoughts	**Boronia** (Bush) for breaking the pattern
Father difficulties of all kinds	**Red Helmet Orchid** (Bush) for a better relationship with the male sex
Obsessive about rules	**Yellow Cowslip Orchid** (Bush) for impartiality and constructiveness

Symptoms	Remedy
Obsessive-compulsive behaviour stemming from sexual abuse or shaming by others	**Pink Monkeyflower** (FES) for courage to take emotional risks with others
Fear related to spiritual or occult phenomena	**Purple Monkeyflower** (FES) for calmness and clarity during spiritual experiences
Addictive mental, emotional and physical patterns	**Forsythia** (Pacific) for transformation, motivation
Indecision	**Pipsissewa** (Pacific) for clearing ambivalence
Feeling unwanted for whatever reason	**Formula Leucantha** (St Germain) for a sense of being nurtured

6
Nervousness and Stammering

In the English language the words 'nerves' and 'nervousness' are a colloquial and somewhat old-fashioned way of describing mental states of anxiety and fear. If you think of yourself as 'a nervous wreck', or that your 'nerves are upset by the least little thing', or that some years ago you suffered from a 'nervous breakdown', try to analyse the experience in more detail before attempting to match that state to specific remedies.

Frequently, nervousness seems to be a learned behaviour. Children sometimes display 'nerves' because a relative did exactly the same when they were growing up. Sometimes we feel very real physical pains in various parts of our body during these times of stress or anxiety. In this case, our state of nervousness is possibly being somatised; in other words, a sense of anxiety is being suppressed in the mind and instead manifests as discomfort in the body.

The mental states described in this book that relate to depression tend to have a cousinly – or more direct – relationship to our early life, and to feelings and events that have since been buried in our subconscious and forgotten.

Case study: Richard
Stammering

Richard was brought to me suffering from uncontrollable stammering, which had started as soon as he could speak. He came from a large family and his mother had a respect for flower essences – she kept a box of Bach remedies at home and had used

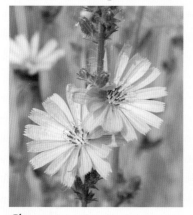

them on several occasions for Richard but without any effect on his stammering. It could be particularly pronounced at school, and on occasions Richard had to be returned to the family for the day when he was quite unable to express himself. Knowing that his mother had explored all the obvious remedies, I adopted the intuitive approach, and with

Chicory

surprise and interest I came up with Bach's **Chicory**.

I was very impressed when I heard later that within two days the stammering had stopped. I sat down to think through what had occurred and, if possible, to discover why. Dr Bach tells us that **Chicory** is a 'type' remedy designed to fine tune people's characters.

Chicory is for those who are very mindful of the needs of others; they tend to be over-full of care for children, relatives, friends ... continually correcting what they consider wrong, and enjoy doing so.

Dr Bach

58

Chicory types desire closeness with those they care about, which has unfortunately led to a more recent association with self-pity, self-love and possessiveness. Richard had a large family, but was rather small within it: he had to make his voice heard. Whether consciously or unconsciously, he discovered that stammering was the answer: everyone had to do the decent thing and stop to listen so that he was heard. When Richard's soul was brought back into alignment by the remedy, he no longer had to demand attention in this way from his family members, and could finally let the stammering go.

Turn to page 202 to find out more about selecting and sourcing these essences.

Treatment

Symptoms	Remedy
Feelings of abandonment resulting in needy or manipulative behaviour	**Chicory** (Bach) for love and care that gives freely to others
Discouragement, doubt, despondency	**Gentian** (Bach) for taking heart and having faith
Fear of known things	**Mimulus** (Bach) for bravery
Alarmed, scared, horror and dread	**Rock Rose** (Bach) for finding the courage to face emergencies
Insistent, wilful, fervent, stressed	**Vervain** (Bach) for quietness and tranquillity
Needing physical and mental renewal	**Olive** (Bach) for rest and support
Out of control energy	**Red Poppy** (Bailey) for finding our true energy and power
Energy dominates	**Yin/Yang Balancer** (Bailey) for balancing the male and female energies

PART TWO: TREATING DIFFERENT FORMS OF DEPRESSION

Symptoms	Remedy
Anger, frustration and sadness of grief	**Yorkshire Fog** (Bailey) for expressing grief, not being entangled by it
Nervous intensity, constant striving	**Black-Eyed Susan** (Bush) for turning inward, slowing down
Excessive worry	**Crowea** (Bush) for peace and calm
Nerves from shyness, fears, phobias	**Dog Rose** (Bush) for confidence and self-belief
Worry over decisions, dithering	**Jacaranda** (Bush) for being decisive and centred
Drained, jaded, burned out	**Macrocarpa** (Bush) for enthusiasm, inner strength, endurance
Nervous problems from over-stimulation or chaotic lifestyle; drug and alcohol abuse	**Morning Glory** (FES) for sparkling vital force; being in touch with natural rhythms
Using addictive substances to numb the nervous system	**Nicotiana** (FES) for inner peace centred in the heart and breath
Feeling and internalising disturbances from outside oneself	**Pink Yarrow** (FES) for appropriate emotional boundaries
Fear related to spiritual or occult phenomena	**Purple Monkeyflower** (FES) for calmness and clarity during spiritual experiences

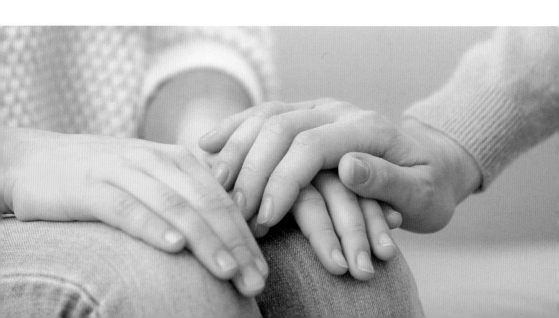

7

Hormonal Depression
(Relating to Puberty, PMT, Fertility, Postnatal Depression, Menopause and Impotence)

Hormones guide us through transitional times in our lives that encompass mental and emotional (as well as physical) changes, which continue over the years. Women typically remain fertile until their mid-forties, at which point the menopause sets in. Men remain fertile until many years later, though testosterone levels do decline gradually with age.

Sometimes these transitioning processes get derailed, often as the result of difficulties in early life, and the free flow of growth and sex hormones may be interrupted without any apparent physical concerns, but leading to various forms of depression, in some cases where the very strong emotions engendered can cause changes to the hormonal process itself.

And around the world, irrespective of culture, a greater occurrence of hormonal depression is reported among women than among men. Social taboo around depression aside, this may well be because of the greater fluctuation of hormones in women's lives than in men's.

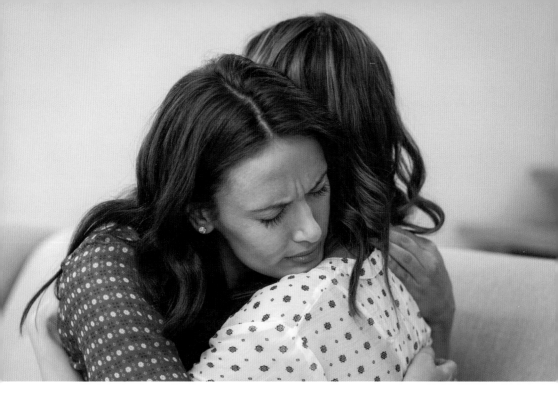

Hormonal depression can start with puberty and can continue in line with the menstrual cycle, followed by an intensification in the 'peri-menopausal' period during the two or three years before the menopause.

Antidepressant medication can be even more often a 'false friend' for this type of depression than with other types, and hormone replacement therapy (HRT) probably brings more relief to women afflicted with conditions of this kind than any other type of prescription medication – though this also comes with its downsides.

As we have seen in earlier chapters, it is my belief that childhood trauma – even prior to birth – is often the cause of depression in later life. Problems experienced in early childhood, so often buried in the detail in our subconscious – such as feeling unwanted, problems during birth, abuse, feeling insecure, or not receiving enough empathy – can be interpreted later in life as reasons for not wanting to reproduce. A war arises: the instinct implanted by Mother Nature is strong and demanding; the contrary urge from our subconscious is equally imperative.

In the invisible conflict that ensues, symptoms of depression can be one outcome. In more severe cases, puberty can be delayed: boys' testicles may fail to descend; girls' periods may start late. Or something like the opposite might occur, as happened in the case of Renata, reported in the case study below.

Puberty

Case study: Renata
Puberty, difficult periods

Renata, a fifteen-year-old girl, had started **puberty** at the age of ten, as had her mother before her, so that it seemed to be something of a genetic condition. She suffered extremely long, drawn-out and **difficult periods**, and her breasts developed early. The relationship between her parents had been deteriorating for a long time; it seemed to be not a question of whether they would split up, but when. Apparently in compensation, her adolescence had started early and strongly. It was as if she were unconsciously saying, 'I will advance into adulthood and relationships and do it properly where my parents have failed'.

But of course mixed messages arose: her early development meant she felt isolated from her peer group; she rounded her shoulders, consciously or unconsciously, in an effort to make her breasts less obvious; and she lost a significant part of her childhood. She was **angry**: with her childhood girlfriends who were amazed at her development; at the boys who reacted to the physical signs of her maturity; at her parents, and at the world in general. She was a thoughtful and accomplished artist at school who found the more academic subjects difficult to engage with, so I first gave her **Vision Quest** from Flower Essences of Fox Mountain to encourage her in her area of greatest talent. This brought her some relief and I followed it up with **Walking out of Patterns** from Dancing Light Orchid Essences. Over a number of months the intensity of her period pains gradually diminished.

Female reproductive issues

A girl moving into puberty is in a vulnerable transitional phase in her life. If during this process she is checked inappropriately, for example by an unwanted sexual advance, she may well be traumatised. And, as we know, the trauma may become locked into the body, damaging her sexual development by interrupting the normal hormonal flow.

Unfortunately, many fertility issues are due to physical conditions that cannot be addressed by flower essences or psychotherapy, for example if surgery has made conception impossible. But I believe that fertility in general, including the IVF process, can be undermined by an unconscious reluctance to conceive. I have sometimes found that women who are struggling to conceive have experienced fundamental difficulties earlier in life, so fundamental that they seriously question, consciously or unconsciously, whether reproducing is worthwhile. If my childhood was so difficult, says the would-be mother, then do I really want to face the prospect of creating life anew? For women at least, the battle is waged most fiercely in their mid-thirties to mid-forties. Nature seems to be ensuring that they address the issues arising from their early lives before they are truly ready to conceive.

Treat depression before trying to conceive

I have observed through my work that conception and a satisfactory birth may become significantly more likely after a period of healing and reflection.

64

Postnatal depression

A vital function of hormones is to facilitate the bond between mother and baby. They act to protect babies in their early days. Mothers are tightly programmed by these hormones to look after their babies, but sometimes the vast changes in hormonal balance during and after pregnancy, plus the exhaustion and stress of giving birth and looking after a baby can lead to postnatal (or post-partum) depression.

More than just the 'baby blues'

Postnatal depression can be physically, emotionally and socially debilitating for the sufferer. The British NHS states that one in ten parents experiences postnatal depression (even fathers!).

Case study: Gillian
Postnatal depression

Gillian had experienced a **difficult first birth** – a non-elective Caesarean – and many weeks later her little boy was still screaming all night, every night. The trauma of the birth and resultant **exhaustion** meant that she **struggled to bond** with her son afterwards. I gave her three Wild Earth Animal Essences:

- ✿ **Letting Go**, a composite that releases feelings, beliefs and actions that no longer serve us
- ✿ **Wild Horse**, which 'nurtures a sense of loving openness, belonging and connection with others' for those with a 'lost heart'
- ✿ **Wolf**, which helps with grounding, and 'nurtures a sense of Divine presence'

These calmed and helped her through those first difficult months, and when she became pregnant with her second baby she was able to put aside the difficult memories of her first child's birth and allow nature to take its course.

Her experience with her second boy was a huge improvement. Their bond developed rapidly and she felt confident and bonded with both children by this point. However, when it became time for her to return to work she found herself feeling exhaustion and grief once more. From the Flower Essence Society I gave her:

- **Splendid Mariposa Lily** to promote a spiritual understanding of mothering
- **Tall Mountain Larkspur**, which encourages one to 'hear, see and act in a greater capacity of soul leadership'

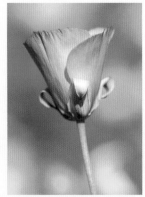

Splendid Mariposa Lily

A month later, although her energy had improved, her **hormonal depression** remained. I followed up with Bach's:

- **Gentian**, which banishes despondency
- **Gorse** to encourage hope

Soon her grief and depression melted away, allowing her to enjoy her life and her motherhood more freely.

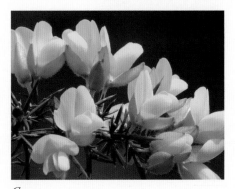

Gorse

66

A post-birth boost

To cover a range of postnatal difficulties, I would recommend Bach's **Gentian** for despondency, **Olive** for exhaustion, **Star of Bethlehem** for shock and **Gorse** for renewed hope.

The treatment section at the end of this chapter features other essences that are helpful for bringing hormonal levels back into balance, while additional essences may help deal with other factors that might be sustaining or contributing to this type of depression.

Returning to work

Many mothers nowadays are faced with returning to work before either they or their babies are ready.

Case study: Carmela
End of maternity leave, anxiety

Carmela came close to a breakdown when the time came for her to return to work after her statutory maternity leave. Her partner had a full-time job away from home so their five-month-old baby girl was cared for by grandparents and a nursery. Carmela's head very clearly wanted her job back, but **her heart said no**.

In fact she did go back to her old job, and I prescribed Bach's **Holly** to support her in this painful situation. I followed it up with Wildflower's **Harmony** to encourage her to be positive and lighten up, and to keep her heart open so that joy could be rekindled. **Harmony**'s components are:

- **Bluebell**, which 'rekindles our connection with nature and our inner wisdom, helps to break through old patterns, provides peace and protection'
- **Celestite**, which reduces stress, anxiety, fear, worry and self-destructive tendencies
- **Purple Foxglove**, which 'enables us to distance ourselves from emotional turmoil' and also encourages communication of the heart
- **Oak**, which balances and grounds the male aspects of our nature and promotes trust
- **Beech**, to balance and ground the female aspects of our nature and promote faith
- **Holly**, which 'encourages us to be positive, keep our hearts open and lighten up when feeling burdened'

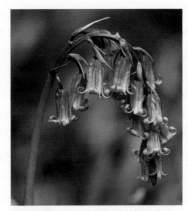

Bluebell

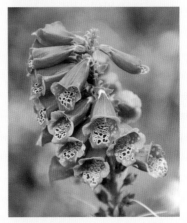

Purple Foxglove

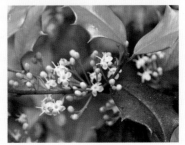

Holly

I also supported her daughter, as flower essences are perfectly safe for children:

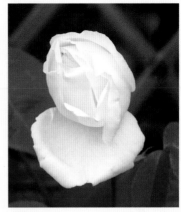

- **Heather**, from Harebell Remedies, which 'gives a subtle boost of courage to accept certain periods of aloneness, feelings of emptiness and lack of certainty'
- **White Rosebud**, to be used with infants 'to help them grow and to keep a sense of heaven on earth'

White Rosebud

Menopause

Usually women experience their menopause during their mid-to-late forties or early fifties, but the effects can reverberate through their lives for years. As ever, mind and body are coupled more tightly than we realise, and whilst many women weather the storm without great inconvenience, some discover unresolved issues during this substantial transition.

Why does the menopause trigger depression?

For those who are subject to depression, the menopause can trigger further depression because there is an aspect of the menopause that can feel like loss.

During the menopause many women feel a strong sense of loss – especially the loss of youth and a perceived loss of conventional attractiveness – which they experience in different ways:

- physical changes, including weight gain
- an increase in facial hair and thinning scalp hair
- loss of fertility
- loss of physical enjoyment in intercourse
- perceived loss of children as they fly the nest around this time

Women who wished to have children but were unable to can experience a strong sense of loss, as can some who consciously decided not to have children.

It seems plausible that some of the well-known symptoms of menopause such as **irritability, insomnia, hot flushes,** and **loss of memory and concentration** may in fact be somatised (or physical) manifestations of depression. Women with unresolved anger issues may suffer particularly fierce hot flushes, or become highly irritable. And perhaps those who have lived most in the mind may be more at risk of loss of memory and concentration than those who allowed themselves to be governed by natural rhythms. But as a general guide, try the following essences:

Hot flushes (anger)

Wild Earth's combination essence called **Healthy Anger, Dagger Hakea** from Australian Bush Flowers, or **Orange Honeysuckle** from Pacific Essences, which might prove particularly appropriate:

> ... for women going through menopause who have directed a lot of energy into birthing and raising their families. When their children leave home they often

feel lost and have no outlet for the expression of their energy... Often this results in a crisis of personal identity and accompanying tension in the physical body. **Orange Honeysuckle** helps us to tap into that place of inner body wisdom and to redirect the energy accordingly.[1]

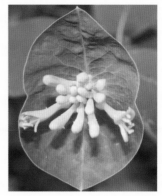

Orange Honeysuckle

Irritability

Ian White from the Australian Bush Flowers might recommend **Black-Eyed Susan**, and Paul Strode of English Wildflowers might opt for his **Harmony** composite essence (detailed on p. 67–69).

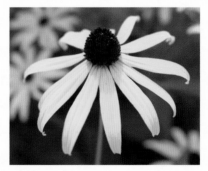

Black-Eyed Susan

Memory and concentration difficulties

Paul Strode of English Wildflowers (see above) would probably recommend the **Harmony** essence. Ian White would select **Isopogon** from Australian Bush Flowers, or his composite essence called **Cognis**. Another Australian composite remedy is **Essence of Clarity** from Living Essences of Australia.

Male reproductive issues

Of course, men have issues with their hormones too. The main British pharmaceutical prescribing guide, the British National Formulary, recognises that erectile dysfunction can originate in the mind. One of the ways in which boys and men can subconsciously acknowledge trauma (especially from early life) is through later impotence. At the crucial moment, testosterone doesn't do its job, and they fulfil their early programming by stifling the next generation.

A range of drugs are available to deal with the symptom superficially, of which Viagra is the best known. But these drugs cannot address a message being sent by the unconscious that has arisen from unaddressed issues.

Addressing the real causes of impotence

I would argue that using flower essences to reach back and rewrite our early programming is a more wholesome way of achieving normal sexual performance than taking Viagra.

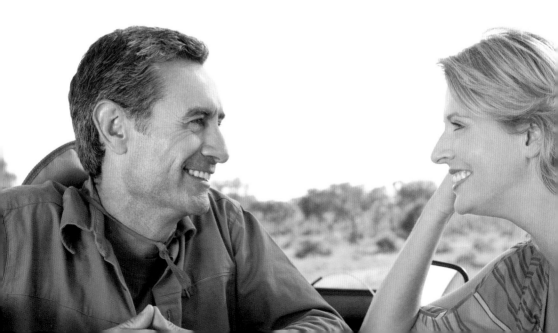

Treatment

Hormonal depression can accompany us, women especially, throughout life from puberty to old age, and there are many remedies that can help along the way.

This is easier to propose than to achieve, however, and it can help enormously to select flower essences that assist what is in effect a process of discovery. At first, essences should help to minimise the worst aspects of a disrupted cycle. Then, as the symptoms are eased, the emphasis should shift towards finding essences that provide the greatest help with our creativity (see Chapter 28).

Remember, each person is different and constantly changing: what works for us at a certain moment will not necessarily be so effective at another time.

Having made some more specific suggestions earlier, here is a larger list for you to browse before you make a decision. Turn to page 202 to find out more about selecting and sourcing these essences.

Symptoms	Remedy
Thoughts of doing dreadful things	**Cherry Plum** (Bach) for calmness and sanity
Discouragement, doubt, despondency	**Gentian** (Bach) for taking heart and having faith
Hopelessness, expectation of suffering	**Gorse** (Bach) for deep and abiding conviction and hope
Jealousy, envy, revenge, anger	**Holly** (Bach) for love that conquers all
Persevering despite difficulties	**Oak** (Bach) for admitting to limitation
Exhausted, lack of strength	**Olive** (Bach) for feeling rested and supported
Worry for others, projecting worry	**Red Chestnut** (Bach) for trusting life
Trauma after a fright or sudden alarm	**Star of Bethlehem** (Bach) for balance and harmony
Dominating, demanding obedience	**Vine** (Bach) for becoming a loving leader and teacher

Symptoms	Remedy
Lack of direction, unfulfilled	**Wild Oat** (Bach) for becoming definite and purposeful
Dissatisfied, bitter, resentful	**Willow** (Bach) for uncomplaining acceptance
Deep conditioned patterns	**Childhood** (Bailey) for dissolving old implanted patterns
Ungrounded from psychic opening	**Thrift** (Bailey) for staying grounded
The stress of major change	**Transition** (Bailey) for making way for the new
Addicted to permanent busyness	**Tree Mallow** (Bailey) for relaxation in the present moment
Not at ease with our sexuality	**Tufted Vetch** (Bailey) for rebalancing our sexual self-image
Unbalanced water energies	**Water** (Bailey) for going with the flow
Lacking intuition and logic	**Yin/Yang Balancer** (Bailey) for harmony and dynamic stillness
Impatience, irritability	**Black-Eyed Susan** (Bush) for slowing down, inner peace
Unresolved mother issues	**Bottlebrush** (Bush) for letting go and moving on
Anger, resentment, and bitterness to those close to you	**Dagger Hakea** (Bush) for forgiveness
Hormonal imbalance	**Fuchsia** (Bush) for rebalancing the hypothalamus
Stale relationships, self-interest	**Gardenia** (Bush) for family bonding and communication
Unresolved father issues	**Red Helmet Orchid** (Bush) for bonding of father with child
Emotional turmoil and rawness	**Red Suva Frangipani** (Bush) for inner peace and strength to cope
Guilt, regret and remorse	**Sturt Desert Rose** (Bush) for courage, being true to self, integrity

Symptoms	Remedy
Non-physical inability to conceive	**She Oak** (Bush) for infertility, PMT, menopausal symptoms
Disembodied feminine self	**Alpine Lily** (FES) for self-assured feminine identity
Struggling to come to terms with the loss of a child	**Bleeding Heart** (FES) for letting go
Grief at menopause	**Borage** (FES) for buoyant courage and optimism
Rejection, from earliest childhood	**Evening Primrose** (FES) for healing painful early emotions
Alienated from mothering role	**Mariposa Lily** (FES) for nurturing maternal consciousness
Conflict between career and home life	**Pomegranate** (FES) for joyful feminine creativity
Bitterness, resentment, stuckness	**Chickweed** (Pacific) for being completely present
PMT/PMS	**Easter Lily** (Pacific) for truth, purity, integrity, honesty
Postnatal depression	**Hooker's Onion** (Pacific) for feeling light-hearted and refreshed
Menopause	**Orange Honeysuckle** (Pacific) for evoking peaceful creativity
Being not doing	**Red Huckleberry** (Pacific) for introspection and regeneration
Misunderstood and out of step	**Wallflower** (Pacific) for attuning to our own inner rhythms
Feeling disconnected, anxious	**Harmony** (Wildflower) for providing a sense of maternal love and support

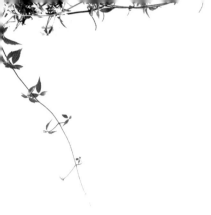

8
Seasonal Affective Disorder (SAD)

SAD has many of the characteristics of general depression. Onset typically occurs in our twenties and thirties, and is reported more often by women than by men.

Symptoms of SAD

These include fatigue, sleepiness, mood swings and food cravings, particularly for carbohydrates and sweet things.

What distinguishes SAD from other kinds of depression is a marked seasonality: the symptoms are normally absent during the summer months and appear with the onset of autumn, continuing until spring brings longer days. In fact, the further we live from the equator, the more likely we are to suffer from the disorder. For example, Americans have reported SAD six times as often in Alaska than in Florida.

Inevitably this has led to the belief that the cause of the affliction is a reduction in the amount of light and/or vitamin D we produce:

the SAD Society recommends regular treatment with a light box to alleviate the symptoms. Perversely, however, a small number of SAD sufferers follow exactly the opposite pattern to their peers. *Their* symptoms come on in summer and abate during the winter months, apparently turning the current theory on its head. As SAD was only isolated as a separate and identifiable disorder in the 1980s, there is clearly room for further investigation into its causation.

The likelihood of SAD following a pattern comparable to more common forms of depression, whereby latent depression is created in the early years by problems of some form, and then brought to the surface in later life by a trigger – in this case a seasonal one – should not be discounted.

Furthermore, SAD does not always occur uniquely as a disorder in itself, but can accompany other illnesses. A number of my clients who have been diagnosed with other illnesses identify the winter as their bad time. One client told me that, of the four times she had been in hospital with bipolar disorder, three of them had been during the run up to Christmas.

Case study: Zahir
SAD, emotional stress

Zahir came to me at the age of 33. His symptoms included back and stomach aches and, as my dowsing uncovered, a musculo-skeletal imbalance. On top of this, of course, he complained of SAD. His **stomach and back aches** had been apparent since the traumatic delivery of his son, who had almost died at birth, and he was under additional emotional stress due to the recent death of his father. He was working extremely hard – indeed the possibility of losing his job seemed to be a contributor to the back pain.

Initially I gave him two essences to relieve his symptoms:

- Bloesem's **Wilde Bertram (Sneezewort)**, which helps you to 'stand on your own two feet and give expression to your thoughts and visions, without having to lean on others'

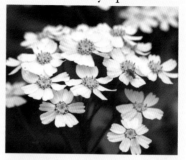

Sneezewort

- The Fox Mountain combination **Vital Balance** (which includes Wild Ginger)

In our third session together he reported that his back pain was continuing to the point where he had been taking anti-inflammatories and painkillers, which in turn brought on distension and stomach pain.

I discovered that he was experiencing an underlying

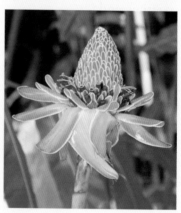

Wild Ginger

ingrained state of fear because of early childhood trauma. He was also feeling **guilt**, perhaps the guilt children often feel when they are neglected ('What is wrong with me?') and perhaps, more recently, because he felt he was not giving enough support to his wife and son owing to his heavy workload. To match and antidote these states I prescribed Wild Earth's:

- **Swan** 'for those who are judgmental of themselves and others'
- **Whale**, which 'calms and clears the mind and allows one to connect with Higher Intelligence'

- 🏵 **Wolf**, which 'encourages right action'

In a later session he reported that his back and stomach pains had significantly decreased, but that he was under pressure from his wife to spend more time at home. I gave him Living Tree's:

- 🏵 **Winged Gold** 'to discover the flowing purpose of our lives'
- 🏵 **Gentle Geisha**, which 'calms the overactive mind'

I believe he did then spend more time with his family and felt less guilt as a consequence. His back pain, stomach aches and the SAD had receded completely by the time we stopped working together, and his vital energy had improved significantly.

Treatment

In most cases it is the underlying emotional states that require confrontation, rather than the symptoms. These emotional states may have been engendered by difficulties that, as in Zahir's case, go back to the very beginning of life. The effect of the essences in shifting the challenging patterns can mean a dramatic improvement in physical ailments as well as in the emotional states themselves.

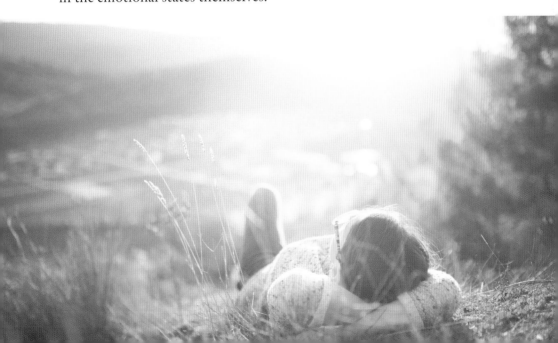

If we ignore the seasonality of SAD, we find that its symptoms are similar to those of other forms of depression, so looking at the essences suggested in any of the earlier chapters may well be appropriate. However, Pacific Essences makes a few remedies which they claim to be particularly helpful for SAD. Turn to page 202 to find out more about selecting and sourcing these essences.

Symptoms	Remedy
SAD – shock, trauma, despair	**Grape Hyacinth** (Pacific) for rebalancing and perspective
SAD – confusion, forgetfulness, despair, depression	**Periwinkle** (Pacific) for remembering and being centred
SAD – resistance	**Snowberry** (Pacific) for acceptance and enthusiasm

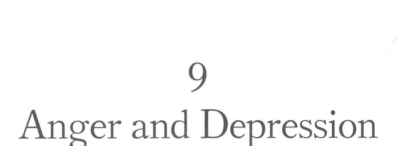

9
Anger and Depression

Anger and depression are intimately linked. Like all our emotions, anger is valuable – there to tell us what we don't like, or to help us to respond powerfully when provoked. However, because it is a very strong emotion, we sometimes struggle to handle our behaviour in response to anger responsibly. Often anger occurs quickly, particularly when a rapid response is called for, but not always – most of us have also experienced slow anger that builds and burns over time.

Because anger is a very forceful emotion, whether fiery or slow-burning, it needs to be expressed outwardly in a conscious way. When not expressed, but frustrated and repressed, it can lead to dejection and states of depression.

The opposite of anger is love

In fact, because love is the strongest emotion of all, it is, ultimately, the opposite of all negative emotion.

Love is quite simply the ground of our being, the place we come from and the place to which we aim to return. When we first arrive on Earth as babies, our mother stands for this love and, when she goes away, we express anger and aggression in order to achieve reunion with her: crying and rage signals our deep distress at the loss we are experiencing. Often our mere perception of the loss of her love produces such anger. And when that anger fails to restore our loss – or is repressed for some reason – we can lapse into mourning, which is indistinguishable from depression in young children.[1]

Frequently this perception of loss, carried over into later life, can produce a cycle of anger and depression. Even small losses in later life can act as triggers to the original, unprocessed loss, and lead to anger and/or depression. This cycle can be repeated throughout life unless and until the original loss is resolved.

Try Holly, Dr Bach's primary anger remedy

Dr Bach described **Holly** as that which protected people 'from everything that was not Universal Love'[2] and which countered all those strong emotions that can distance us from it: **jealousy**, **distrust**, **rage**, **envy** and **hatred**. **Holly** works by moving us back towards our key source of love – found no longer in our mother, but deep within us.

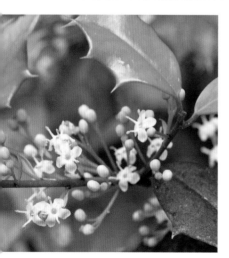

For the first seven years of life, parents provide the love and nurture their children need. After that, children gradually grow and learn to take on these functions for themselves, developing enough inner love to sustain, in due course, the next generation.

The late Steve Johnson, of the Alaskan Flower Essence Project, even recommended that we recite this affirmation when taking his remedy, **Blue Elf Viola**.

Holly

I understand the seeds of my anger and release them into love. What I feel, I can heal.[3]

Steve Johnson, AFEP

We can say again that anger is a valuable emotion: a cause of anger arises, we recognise it, we express the anger rightfully, and then we move on. Just as a head of steam builds up in a boiler, is vented through the safety valve, and normal functioning resumes. And if we can understand the spring from which the anger rose we have come a long way towards managing it.

Bottled-up anger takes a lot of energy to suppress, and Steve Johnson tells us how **Blue Elf Viola** can help us release it responsibly:

The **Blue Elf Viola** essence helps us dissipate the layers of protective energy we have built up around our anger and frustrations, so that we may gain a better understanding of the core feelings at the root of these emotions and allow

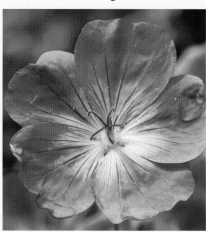

them to be released. The essence of **Blue Elf Viola** brings the energy and understanding of the heart into this process, enabling us to express our anger in a clear but non-violent way, forgive those responsible (including ourselves), and bring the whole emotional cycle to completion.[4]

Blue Elf Viola

Case study: Frederick
Anger, parental relationships

Frederick is a good example of a person I worked with who had long-suppressed anger issues with his father. Interestingly, it seemed that his father was a well-meaning man who intended to love his children, but could not control his own anger – repeating the cycle from his own severe upbringing. Frederick's story serves to show how, unless we take time to heal our hurt, inappropriately expressed anger can be continued down the generations.

Before I even met Frederick I had to make up a 'holding' remedy for him and recommend he seek further help as he was feeling suicidal. I gave him:

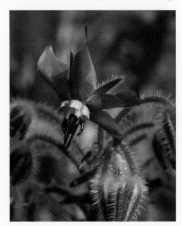

Borage

- **Komkommerkruid (Borage)** (Bloesem Remedies)
- **Grieving** (Fox Mountain)

These two remedies strengthen the heart and restore lost faith. When we did get together, I found that he was taking two antidepressants, two diabetes drugs, something to lower his cholesterol and a blood thinner. Not surprisingly, his **energy was very low** and he was concerned about this level of medication. He told me that his father had been particularly hard on him when he was a child, insisting that he and his brothers undertook what seemed like an endless round of chores, leaving them with no free time. This was exacerbated because he had a wild younger brother, a proper black sheep, who was extremely hard to handle at home and at school. Frederick insisted on standing up for him, protecting him from his **father's anger**, and sometimes claiming the brother's escapades for his own.

The remedies I gave him were:

- 🏵 **Black-Eyed Susan** (Fox Mountain) which is specifically for anger, frustration, bitterness and irritability
- 🏵 **Engelwortel (Angelica)** (Bloesem), which 'strengthens the ability to experience loving spiritual forces in your life and work'.

This helped initially to soothe Frederick's anger and frustration about his father's behaviour towards him. But then, in a later session, the issue of his relationship with his own son came up: they lived in a modern open-plan home and worked almost on top of one another, and Frederick admitted he could be highly critical of his son's work and behaviour. Although he, Frederick, abhorred his father's angry behaviour, this was the only model he'd had in his life for how to manage **father-son relationships**. Frederick was well aware that he was replicating his father's behaviour, albeit in a milder form. For this I gave him:

- 🏵 **Zevenblad (Ground Elder)** (Bloesem) for 'difficulty in assimilating everything that you meet, especially old restrictions and old emotions, which keep you stuck in certain patterns'

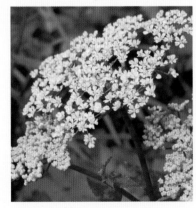

Ground Elder

❀ **Rock Spring** (AFEP) 'to help us find our way through seemingly insurmountable obstacles with infinite patience and never-ending trust'

After this, Frederick started to feel significantly better and decided to take more responsibility and spend more time with his children. We continued to work together for some months and, by the time we stopped, his energy level had risen substantially, his work-life balance was improved, and he was beginning to reduce his medication. Interestingly, Frederick's own father, now 83, had also begun to reconsider his behaviour and become more friendly and supportive towards his sons.

The second element to this case study, that of addiction, is addressed in Chapter 4: while Frederick's father's former harsh treatment of him gave Frederick every reason to be angry, my dowsing suggested that his condition had a strong iatrogenic component – in other words, he had been taking **too much medication** for too long and it was doing him harm. Essences work with the whole system, so when that system has been altered in some way by taking drugs, pharmaceutical or otherwise, the therapist will select essences to respond to both the primary problem and the effects of the medication.

Treatment

Here are some essences that help to deal with inappropriate or uncontrollable anger, but do keep an open mind and browse other treatment lists for ideas to address the underlying causes of anger issues. Turn to page 202 to find out more about selecting and sourcing these essences.

Symptoms	Remedy
Expressing anger violently and uncontrollably	**Blue Elf Viola** (AFEP) for understanding one's anger, and the expression of forgiveness
Jealousy, envy, revenge, anger	**Holly** (Bach) for love conquering all
Irritated by constraints, quick to anger, tense, impatient	**Impatiens** (Bach) for gentleness and forgiving
Deeply held anger leading to bitterness	**Willow** (Bach) for uncomplaining acceptance and overcoming resentment
Unstable fire energies	**Anger and Frustration** (Bailey) for balancing energies and avoiding overreaction
Anger and resentment	**Holly Leaf** (Bailey) for letting go of pent-up anger
Impatience, irritability	**Black-Eyed Susan** (Bush) for slowing down, inner peace
Anger, resentment, and bitterness to those close to you	**Dagger Hakea** (Bush) for forgiveness
Fear of anger	**Dog Rose** (Bush) for confronting our fears
Fear of loss of control	**Dog Rose of the Wild Forces** (Bush) for emotional balance and calmness
Anger, hatred, aggression, envy, jealousy	**Mountain Devil** (Bush) for opening up to unconditional love
Repressed anger	**Black-Eyed Susan** (FES) for bringing anger to awareness
Easily upset, moody and irritable	**Chamomile** (FES) for restoring calm, serenity, balance
Deep-seated anger, hyper-emotional	**Fuchsia** (FES) for expressing intense feelings
Expectation of hostility from others, paranoia	**Oregon Grape** (FES) for positive expectation of good will from others
Projecting hostility to avoid intimacy	**Poison Oak** (FES) for the ability to be in close contact with others

Symptoms	Remedy
Fear of anger	**Scarlet Monkeyflower** (FES) for recognising and transforming anger
Verbal aggression and hostility	**Snapdragon** (FES) for emotionally balanced verbal communication
Self-anger around abortion, miscarriage, birth and sexuality	**Candystick** (Pacific) for transforming frustration
Bitterness, resentment and unavailability	**Chickweed** (Pacific) for being present, available and responsive
Abuse, abandonment, psychic, emotional or physical assault	**Nootka Rose** (Pacific) for expressing love of life, laughter and joy
The anger of frustrated creativity	**Orange Honeysuckle** (Pacific) for inner direction and expressing creativity
Anger associated with inability to commit	**Pearly Everlasting** (Pacific) for commitment, devotion, service
Poisonous thoughts and attitudes, resentment	**Plantain** (Pacific) for cleansing and purification
Grudges, resentment	**Salal** (Pacific) for forgiveness

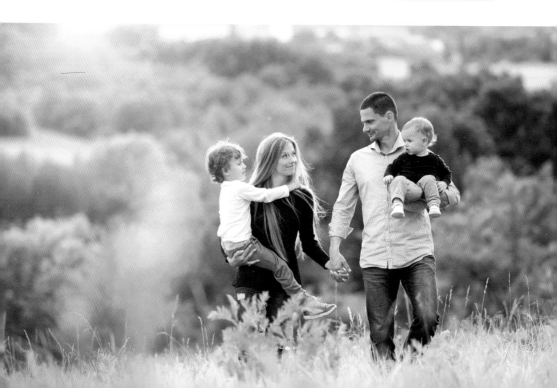

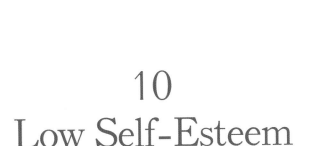

10
Low Self-Esteem

In my view, the most striking characteristic of depressives is a negative one; an absence of built-in self-esteem.[1]

Anthony Storr

A lack of self-esteem seems to be a central feature of many kinds of depression. The psychotherapist and writer Anthony Storr suggested that this might arise from how parents regard their children, which makes perfect sense to me. In my experience, this sense of a lack of self-worth seems to come about by being undervalued and criticised as a child.

One personal example of this is my first wife, who was warmly anticipated as a baby, but then totally failed to please when she turned out to be a girl. Her mother was one of four sisters – no brothers – born to a sporting lion, a famous cricketer of his day, who placed an enormous premium on boys in the family. Valerie was not exactly neglected by her mother, but undervalued. Sporting achievements were considered of central importance in the family, and she concentrated on them and strove to please, but her efforts were never seen as remotely adequate, and her mother consistently derided her level of play on the school sports field.

When children experience persistent criticism, they consider it a form of education, like any other. They internalise these negative views, place a low worth upon themselves, and carry that understanding into later life. Without help, that feeling cannot be eradicated. And in Valerie's case her lack of self-esteem predominantly expressed itself in these three ways:

1. She undervalued her intellectual and academic capability and potential
2. She had a great lack of confidence regarding love
3. On the balancing side, she had a powerful drive to succeed with any project she undertook

> Learning to cope more effectively with life and with one's own temperament will not be brought about by drugs; and although temporary alleviation can be affected by their prescription, continued long-term use is seldom justified, and may actually be harmful, since it tends to blunt the patient's sensibilities, and prevents him from coming to terms with reality.[2]
>
> *Anthony Storr*

My solution would naturally be to work with essences as well as psychotherapy. Sometimes a well chosen essence can banish the problem almost indefinitely, but in general I would be inclined to echo Storr's claim. I think depression remains a part of you, and a useful one at that, able to act as a salutary reminder when it does recur that somehow your life has run off its true path.

The self-criticism we learn from our parents can, within reason, be harnessed to good use in developing our own discrimination – and energy. For example, we rebuilt a derelict house in two-and-a-half years – including adding another storey. Without Valerie's drive and critical decisiveness, the project would never have started, let alone finished and we gained a lot of fun and satisfaction along the way.

Amanda's story below serves to illustrate the intuitive rationale, if I may put it that way, behind the essences we can sometimes select.

Case study: Amanda
Low confidence and energy

Amanda's reason for coming to see me was that her son had just gone to university and she was missing him a great deal. Her energy level was low. She came from a family where depression – even suicide – was common. She was born with a cyst on her liver, and apparently both she and her mother had experienced difficult births. When she was eight years old her father had 'disappeared' for a period. Her relationship with him had been angry and very difficult ever since, and this seemed to have affected all her later relationships with men.

Surprising myself, I selected **Stepping Ahead Now** from Dancing Light Orchid Essences ('the canvas is ready to receive your brush strokes: step ahead now') for her. Usually, as I have said, when I am working with anger, low confidence and depression, I would first select essences that operated directly on those blockages. **Stepping Ahead Now** pointed her in a direction where she could creatively shape herself rather than raking over the past. My instinct was that this kind of action would be more likely to energise her. The essence worked well, and by the time we next met she felt that her energy had risen significantly.

Now, however, she was feeling **overwhelmed** by her stressful teaching job; she felt tired, in need of approval and was experiencing recurrent anger. All this suggested that it was high time to focus on her **relationship with her father**. I dowsed Living Tree's orchid essences and selected:

- **Just Me**, 'for children who have not felt loved'
- **Golden Radiance**, 'for developing a spiritual perspective on everyday life'

I saw her again a few months later and she felt that her self-esteem had improved and her anger had reduced.

Treatment

Of course, psychotherapy is Storr's own solution, though he does not claim that it can always completely eliminate depression.

Dr Bach's **Beech** is frequently used to treat low self-esteem.

Being overly critical

The problem for the Beech person is a lack of self-worth. Those who do not value themselves find it hard to value and honour others.

Julian Barnard

Beech helps to bring people back to being 'tolerant, lenient and understanding of the different ways each individual and all things are working to their own final perfection'.[3] Barnard believes that Beeches act rather like critical austere sentinels (certain types of parent), refusing to tolerate any way of thinking other than their own.

Beech

To experience fully the tranquillity of the Beech tree, stand in a Beech wood. Here the tall, smooth trunks rise like slender pillars to the vaulting leaf canopy ...

So complete is the high roof's delicate tracery of branches that other plants are starved of light. At the woodland edge, brambles, hollies and hazels may survive, but even here the low sweeping branches of the Beech trees close out the sun. In the Beech remedy state, a person becomes **isolated, lonely and cut off from others.**[4]

Australian Bush flower essence maker Ian White regards a lack of self-esteem, self-worth and self-confidence as being fundamental to the human condition.[5] His primary remedy is called **Five Corners**, which promotes a **love and acceptance of self**, and a celebration of one's own beauty. Red is the colour antidote, he says, to low self-esteem. Turn to page 202 to find out more about selecting and sourcing these essences.

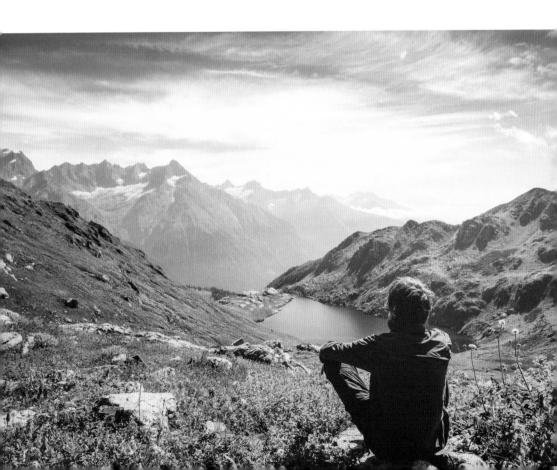

Symptoms	Remedy
Intolerant, critical of ourselves and others	**Beech** (Bach) for seeing more good in the world
Anxious to serve, weak, dominated	**Centaury** (Bach) for serving others from a feeling of self-worth
Distrust of self and intuition; easily led and misguided	**Cerato** (Bach) for strength to follow your inner guidance
Preoccupation with personal suffering	**Heather** (Bach) for tranquillity and kinship with all life
Expecting failure; lacking confidence and will to succeed	**Larch** (Bach) for confidence in your creative abilities
Disempowered, often dominated, unable to assert oneself, sometimes over-aggressive	**Self-esteem composite** (Bailey) for discovering your innate strength and wisdom
Disliking oneself, feeling rotten inside, sinful, unworthy	**Bluebell** (Bailey) for unlocking your hidden potential, blossoming inside
Blocked-off self love	**Butterbur** (Bailey) for realising your essential goodness
Lacking self-confidence, uncertain	**Hawkweed** (Bailey) for feeling more at home in the world
Surrounded by negative conditioning	**Moss** (Bailey) for seeing that we are only frightened by our fears
Feeling trapped by the authoritarian power of others	**Pine Cones** (Bailey) for recognising your own authority
Trying to live up to the expectations of others	**Witch Hazel** (Bailey) for taking your 'mission' in life rather less seriously
Low self-esteem, guilt, shyness, lack of conviction, victim mentality	**Confid composite** (Bush) for taking responsibility for your life, confidence, personal power, true to self
Lack of confidence associated with fear and shyness	**Dog Rose** (Bush) for confidence, self-belief, courage, ability to embrace life more fully
Sabotaging your goals and dreams through believing you do not deserve them	**Five Corners** (Bush) for self-worth, self-love, self-esteem, self-confidence

94

Symptoms	Remedy
Victim mentality, complaining, bitterness, poverty consciousness	**Southern Cross** (Bush) for personal power, taking responsibility, positivity
Guilt, regret and remorse, low self-esteem	**Sturt Desert Rose** (Bush) for courage, conviction, being true to self, integrity
Low self-worth, self-deprecating	**Buttercup** (FES) for knowing your true worth to others
Feeling unloved or unwanted due to trauma, abuse or neglect in early childhood	**Evening Primrose** (FES) for awareness and healing of painful emotions absorbed from parents
Insecurity in relationships and reaching out to others, resulting in social barriers	**Mallow** (FES) for confidence in social situations
Distorted or vacillating sense of self, low self-esteem or arrogance	**Sunflower** (FES) for unique individuality
Lack of vitality in expression, inability to be assertive or to speak clearly	**Trumpet Vine** (FES) for strong, vital speaking and self-expression out of inner self-confidence
Overwhelmed, frustrated, stuck, dense, heavy	**Hooker's Onion** (Pacific) for feeling light-hearted and refreshed, nurturing creativity
Negative sense of self, worthlessness	**Indian Pipe** (Pacific) for self-respect and respect for others
Loss of identity, anger	**Orange Honeysuckle** (Pacific) for creatively redirecting energy
Indecisiveness	**Pipsissewa** (Pacific) for clearing ambivalence, decisiveness
Fear and restriction	**Snowdrop** (Pacific) for letting go, having fun, feeling delight, release
Feeling small, self-loathing	**Vanilla Leaf** (Pacific) for affirmation and acceptance of oneself

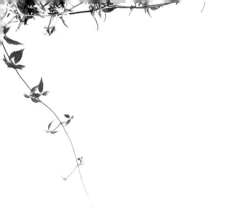

11
Emotional and Physical Stress

Stress shows itself in many ways and therefore has no all-encompassing antidote. If I am feeling overwhelmed by events or having too much to do, **Elm** usually calms me – a stress remedy if ever there was one – but I would not expect to be experiencing physical pain at this point. The remedy will always be different according to the particular needs of each individual. For example, even the burden of choosing can lead to stress. Among the Pacific Essences, **Pipsissewa** is about making the right choice. Sabina Pettitt, who makes these essences, writes, 'If you follow the path that leads to peace of mind and comfort in your heart, it will always be the right choice for you.' And conversely, choosing the wrong path may lead to pain and discomfort.

I do much of my work within a busy cranial osteopathy practice where the pain of stress is encountered on a daily basis. Often the physical pain that osteopaths know well how to treat is recognised as having an emotional origin – and the client is directed to me. The case study below is one of those cases.

Case study: Yvonne
Stress, physical pain

Yvonne arrived with **extreme pain in her neck and shoulder** owing to inflammation from the nerve bundles in the area. The skin there was too painful to touch, and although the painkillers she was taking didn't fully numb the pain they at least enabled her to sleep. She had experienced discomfort for most of her life in that area, although she had only felt this intensity of pain for the past few days, during which she had found herself sobbing for hours at a stretch.

I discovered that from childhood Yvonne had developed deep **issues around intimacy and mistrust**. Now she was faced with a hard choice to make between her lucrative job on the one hand and charitable work she felt committed to on the other. Her yin and yang (yin the feminine and yang the masculine principle, broadly speaking) were out of balance. She initially took away with her:

- **Vine** (Bach) for 'selfless service'[1]
- **Swan** (Wild Earth) 'for expanding one's capacity to acknowledge and accept one's own goodness and beauty'

Three weeks later she was so changed that I failed to recognise her in the waiting room. There was still some discomfort, but the crisis had passed. Her yin and yang were still in need of balancing, however, and she still had to decide between the two jobs. I gave Yvonne:

- **Air** (White Light), which 'produces a sensation of feeling light, easy and carefree'
- **Squirrel** (Wild Earth), which supports us 'in finding a dynamic integration of work and play'

On the surface, **Pipsissewa** would have relieved Yvonne's pain because it would have helped to resolve a question of choice. But something else, it seemed, was needed to work at a deeper level. Physical conditions frequently take some time to shift because they are often the outcome of longstanding imbalance and disturbance in other domains of the body.

Feeling light, easy and carefree

The message from the White Light **Air** essence – feeling light, easy and carefree – sums up the collective overall aim of flower essences. When our burdens are lifted, we can find relief.

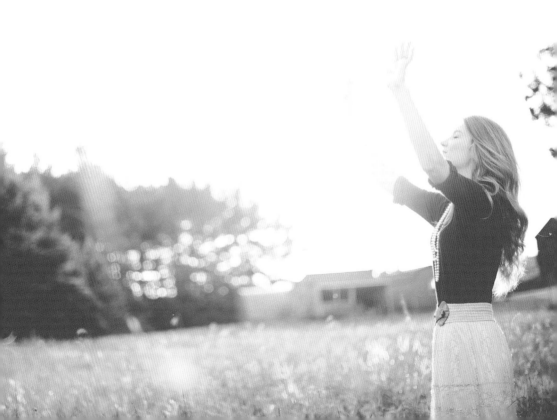

Treatment

Before we move on to suggested essences, we should remember that a certain amount of stress in our lives can be desirable and helpful. Stress drives us out of bed in the morning and encourages us to carry out our proper work, whatever that may be. Without that basic level of stress we run the risk of becoming lazy, which is not the same as living peacefully. Getting the balance in our lives right is one of the fine arts of living. Turn to page 202 to find out more about selecting and sourcing these essences.

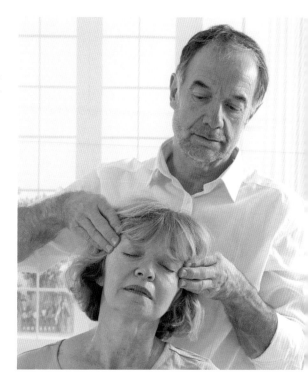

Symptoms	Remedy
Fear that stress will lead to breakdown and loss of control	**Cherry Plum** (Bach) for calmness and sanity
Overwhelmed by responsibility, taking on too much	**Elm** (Bach) for the strength to perform your duty
Extreme stress	**Five Flowers (Rescue Remedy)** (Bach) for bringing balance, especially as a first step
Impatience, frustration, irritation, trying to go too fast	**Impatiens** (Bach) for gentleness and forgiving
Trauma after a fright or sudden alarm	**Star of Bethlehem** (Bach) for balance and harmony
Over-enthusiasm and extremism, leading to nervous breakdown or depletion	**Vervain** (Bach) for quiet and tranquillity

Symptoms	Remedy
Exerting harsh or extreme control over children	**Vine** (Bach) for recognition of the individuality of others
Emotional stress of an overly tense mind	**Fuji Cherry** (Bailey) for encouraging the mind and body to relax
Seeing the world as a threatening place	**Heath Bedstraw** (Bailey) for relaxing and trusting our environment
Being spaced out, uprooted by the forces around us	**Ivy** (Bailey) for being strongly grounded in the world and at ease
The stress of an overactive mind	**Tranquillity** (Bailey) for finding peace within the storms of everyday life
Busyness or its opposite: inertia	**Tree Mallow** (Bailey) for regenerating our drive from a relaxed state of mind
Stress of constantly feeling rushed	**Black-Eyed Susan** (Bush) for knowing how and when to stop and rest
Constant and repetitive thoughts	**Boronia** (Bush) for clarity, serenity, creative visualisation
Always over-committed, no time for self, impatient, rushing, worried	**Calm and Clear combi** (Bush) for finding your own time and space, winding down, relaxing and having fun, calmness, peace
Temporary loss of drive, enthusiasm and excitement	**Dynamis combi** (Bush) for renewing passion for life, harmonising vital forces
Tendency to give up when over-stressed	**Kapok Bush** (Bush) for willingness, application, 'give it a go', persistence
Overwork, burnout, misuse of creativity	**Aloe Vera** (FES) for creative activity integrated with life-energy
Emotional tension stored throughout body, especially in musculature	**Dandelion** (FES) for dynamic physical energy, inner ease in work and play
Paralysis in solar plexus due to fear, stage fright	**Garlic** (FES) for resilient and vital response to life
Nervous tension leading to depletion and exhaustion, insomnia	**Lavender** (FES) for spiritual sensitivity, highly refined awareness intact with bodily health

100

Symptoms	Remedy
Stressful situations	**Goatsbeard** (Pacific) for power to visualise yourself into a state of deep relaxation
Traumatic stress, emotional or physical	**Grape Hyacinth** (Pacific) for balance and perspective
Overwhelm, frustration	**Hooker's Onion** (Pacific) for feeling light-hearted, nurturing creativity
Indecision	**Pipsissewa** (Pacific) for decisiveness, clearing ambivalence

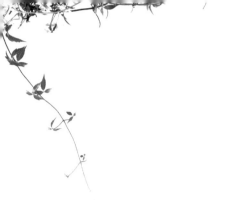

12
Insomnia

Our normal sleep patterns are habitual. We gradually move into a period of deep sleep during the night, which is then succeeded by a period of lighter sleep that heralds our awakening a few hours later. However, if there is any interruption to the rhythm of our daily life that triggers our adrenaline to a degree where it cannot be easily switched off again, the fight-or-flight reaction kicks in and prevents us from drifting off. Or we are granted a period of more or less easy sleep at the beginning of the night, followed by an early awakening once we move into the period of lighter sleep. In extreme cases this early rising becomes the new pattern.

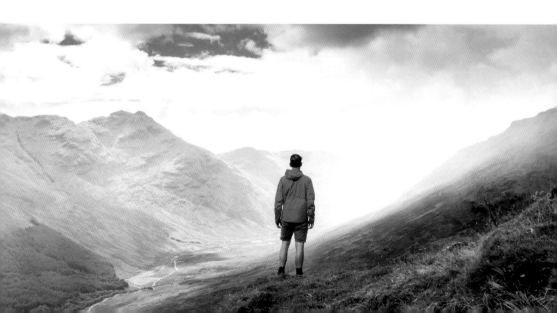

Sometimes the trigger is simple **overwhelm** or **exhaustion**: we have taken on what our bodies and minds perceive as 'too much'. Often a **holiday** can help to break the pattern, or an overwhelm remedy such as Bach's **Elm** brings our reaction to our busy lives back into balance. Turn to Chapter 13 for ways to treat different types of exhaustion.

Occasionally, however, the problem goes deeper. If your habitual pattern in life is to control or attempt to control events, **losing control of situations** you would expect to manage can be deeply stressful and worrying: adrenaline is turned on but cannot be turned off, and insomnia can take over. In these situations try remedies which deal with **anxiety** (Chapter 3) or **stress** (Chapter 11), and if they prove to be unhelpful, seek further advice.

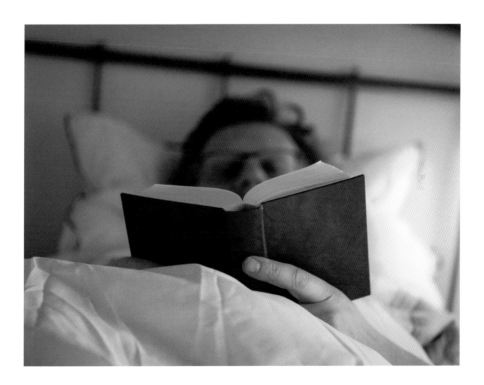

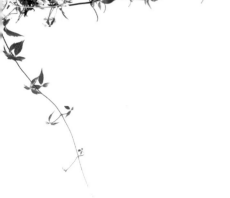

13
Exhaustion

Fatigue, tiredness and exhaustion come about for various different reasons:

- ✿ The deep exhaustion and constant tiredness that grips you after a long struggle with worry, illness or grief may call for Bach's **Olive** remedy[1]
- ✿ To treat burnout following the overuse of creative forces, **Aloe Vera** (FES) can bring life forces to the heart centre[2]
- ✿ For overcoming 'the emotional and physical exhaustion that comes with the long-term care of others or for the burnout of professional health workers',[3] try **Alpine Mint Bush** (Bush)

What seems clear in considering the many and varied states of extreme fatigue is that they can very easily be mistaken for generalised depression.

With cases such as these, I find that it is almost always necessary to go beyond the superficial symptoms and understand something of the client's history before choosing an appropriate essence. I do not have a clear-cut case study to illustrate exhaustion, but I hope the following notes on essences will light your imagination to finding a suitable remedy as you search within yourself. Turn to page 202 to find out more about selecting and sourcing these essences.

Treatment

Symptoms	Remedy
Taking on too much responsibility, overwhelmed by tasks assumed	**Elm** (Bach) for joyous service, faith and confidence to complete your task
Feeling too tired to face the tasks of the day	**Hornbeam** (Bach) for dynamic involvement in life's tasks, steady state of energy
Pushing oneself, even when exhausted	**Oak** (Bach) for balanced strength, accepting limits
Complete depletion of mind and body, fatigue from overwork, physical stress or illness	**Olive** (Bach) for feeling rested and supported, rejuvenation of life force
Nervous exhaustion from extreme or fanatical lifestyle	**Vervain** (Bach) for moderation, quiet and tranquillity
Repetitive circular thoughts prevent sleep	**White Chestnut** (Bach) for a calm clear mind and tranquil disposition
Resignation due to a long lingering illness	**Wild Rose** (Bach) for spirit of joy and adventure
Mental and emotional exhaustion of caregivers	**Alpine Mint Bush** (Bush) for revitalisation, joy, renewal
Emotional exhaustion of over-committed, on-the-go people	**Black-Eyed Susan** (Bush) for the ability to turn inward and be still, slowing down
Physical exhaustion, burnout	**Macrocarpa** (Bush) for enthusiasm, inner strength
Fatigue, exhaustion stemming from low blood-sugar levels	**Peach-flowered Tea Tree** (Bush) for taking responsibility for your health
Emotional exhaustion arising from a difficult relationship	**Red Suva Frangipani** (Bush) for feeling calm and nurtured, having strength to cope
Totally drained, exhausted and at the end of your tether	**Waratah** (Bush) for courage, tenacity, adaptability, strong faith
Overwork, burnout, misuse of creativity	**Aloe Vera** (FES) for creative activity integrated with life-energy

105

Symptoms	Remedy
Blockage of creative vitality, fatigue and lacklustre performance	**Indian Paintbrush** (FES) for lively, energetic creativity, exuberant artistic activity
Nervous exhaustion often accompanied by sexual depletion	**Lady's Slipper** (FES) for higher purpose aligned with daily work
Nervous tension leading to depletion and exhaustion, insomnia	**Lavender** (FES) for spiritual sensitivity, highly refined awareness intact with bodily health
Hyperactivity of mental forces leading to extreme fatigue	**Nasturtium** (FES) for glowing vitality, radiant warmth
Mental fatigue, lethargic thinking	**Peppermint** (FES) for mindful and wakeful clarity
Deep melancholia that invades the body, feeling of wasting away, deterioration	**Yerba Santa** (FES) for the capacity to express a full range of human emotions, especially pain and sadness
Fatigue, limitation, shyness, tongue-tied	**Bluebell** (Pacific) for expressing your own uniqueness
Self-destruction	**Forsythia** (Pacific) for transformation, motivation
Weariness, abuse, abandonment	**Nootka Rose** (Pacific) for expressing love of life, laughter and joy

14
Psychological Trauma

Trauma in the medical sense can refer to a wound or an injury – think of a hospital trauma unit; but as a psychiatric term it means an emotional shock so severe that it can underlie and give rise to mental disorder of some kind. Obviously trauma – mental, emotional or physical – can occur at any time of life and ideally should be treated as soon as possible by seeking medical help, but underlying childhood trauma habitually causes the kind of difficulties that my clients are experiencing.

We 'forget' traumatic times

The traumatic events often happened long ago and we buried the hurt and continued our life, growth and development despite it, yet remained subconsciously deeply influenced by it.

These kinds of difficulties, which may hamper us in various ways and thereby deplete our energy, are the most difficult to detect: they lie at the roots of our personality and we are often unaware of them. Indeed, we unwittingly keep them hidden. It is only when we engage in types of therapy such as **psychotherapy** or **flower essence therapy** that we sometimes uncover them – something apparently Freud was the first to recognise.

What is the reason for this resistance to healing? We take a lot of time and trouble to build our personality; we or others may find it hard to live with, but it has been stress-tested. We know our way of dealing with things works because despite all our problems we are still here to prove that it does, so we are therefore reluctant to let it be changed by any form of therapy. Incidentally, this is the reason why children, animals and plants respond so readily to flower essences compared to mature humans: the former have not put up the adaptive, protective façades that the latter usually prove so capable of building.

Find the courage to talk about it

To help us move forward and become unstuck, our traumas need to be aired, otherwise we will continue to live in pain.

Scilla's story includes severe traumas in youth, and shows the essences working alongside some strong medication.

Case study: Scilla
Severe depression and anxiety, childhood trauma

Scilla came to see me, aged 57, and suffering from severe depression. She was taking two anti-epileptic drugs and a painkiller. Her vital energy level was low. She had been 'put out for fostering' as a child, where she was **abused**, and had also suffered from tuberculosis. She had been troubled by acute **claustrophobia** for much of her life, and following a stroke several years ago she had experienced petit mal epilepsy. More recently, she had also been suffering from painful peripheral neuropathy – a disease affecting the nerves, which impairs sensation, movement, gland or organ function.

At her first session I noted that her underlying state seemed to be **anxiety**, so I gave her:

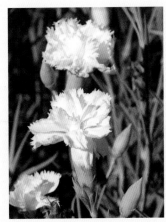

- **White Carnation** (Petite Fleur), which 'reduces wilfulness, increases willpower'
- **Wild Oats** (Petite Fleur) which 'develops sense of humour'. I suspect it relates to Dr Bach's **Wild Oat**, his remedy for creativity

White Carnation

A few days before her second session she had suffered a transient ischaemic (blood circulatory) attack but, nonetheless, her energy seemed to have improved a little. I selected:

- **Death Camas** (Pacific), which 'alleviates stress and worry in times of transition'
- **Red Huckleberry** (Pacific) for 'the power of nourishment and regeneration contained in hibernation'
- The sea essence, **Staghorn Algae** (Pacific), to 'hold a sense of self amidst turbulence and confusion'

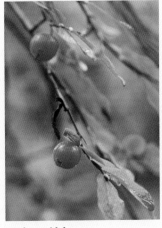

Although her medication continued throughout the process of her treatment with me, and despite difficulties during the previous few weeks, her energy level increased significantly and she was feeling more positive.

Red Huckleberry

Treatment

Some of the most noteworthy points about psychological trauma are its range across all levels – mental, emotional and physical – and its immediacy. Trauma tends to occur suddenly, and, if possible, it is best treated in the same manner – both by seeking medical help and through supporting therapies.

Rescue Remedy

The world's best known flower remedy is a combination of Bach flowers for trauma of all kinds called variously **Rescue Remedy** (Dr Bach's original name for it), **Five Flower remedy** (Healing*herbs*) and other names depending on the maker. It includes **Cherry Plum**, **Clematis**, **Impatiens**, **Rock Rose** and **Star of Bethlehem**, and in combination this remedy can deal with a wide range of shock, whether physical, emotional or mental. It is the one bottle that I carry with me at almost all times.

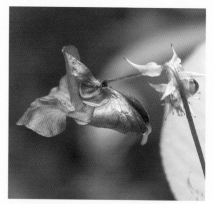

Impatiens

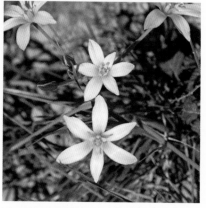

Star of Bethlehem

The Australian Bush Flower range includes **Emergency Essence**, which is a combination of Bush flowers produced with the same idea of an antidote to all kinds of shock and trauma, and the Bailey **Shock and Trauma** composite formula was developed with the same intention. Turn to page 202 to find out more about selecting and sourcing these essences.

Symptoms	Remedy
Panic, disorientation, loss of consciousness, acute trauma or pain	**Five Flowers (Rescue Remedy)** (Bach) for calmness and stability in any emergency or time of stress
Shock or trauma, either recent or from a past experience	**Star of Bethlehem** (Bach) for unity with deepest part of the Self, sense of inner divinity and wholeness
For indecisive, scattered people, underachievers	**Wild Oat** (Bach) for showing us how we can serve, by finding our true vocation or calling
Sudden or long-term shock or trauma	**Shock and Trauma composite** (Bailey) for grounding, ease and comfort, and detachment
Being ungrounded following a shock	**Ivy** (Bailey) for solidly rooting us in the present moment
Disrupted healing process after trauma	**Scabious** (Bailey) for restoring the healing process and bringing perspective
Disruption of the body's energies following shock or trauma	**Star of Bethlehem** (Bailey) for releasing the effects of shock and trauma to the whole system
Panic, distress, fear, inability to cope	**Emergency Essence** (Bush) for calmness and the ability to cope
Terror from nightmares or psychic attack	**Grey Spider Flower** (Bush) for faith, calm, courage
Deep ancient psychic wound	**Pink Mulla Mulla** (Bush) for deep spiritual healing, trusting and opening up

Symptoms	Remedy
Past or present shock or trauma	**Arnica** (FES) for maintaining connection with ego forces during trauma, healing past trauma
Deeply shattering or destructive experiences	**Echinacea** (FES) for core integrity and immunity, maintaining a strong sense of Self
Violation or abuse which leads to emotional closure and profound soul shame	**Pink Monkeyflower** (FES) for courage to take emotional risks with others
Loss of a sense of inner responsibility for your own healing	**Self-Heal** (FES) for recuperative healing from shock
Pelvic tension attributable to trauma	**Candystick** (Pacific) for releasing blocked energy around abortion, miscarriage, birth, sexuality
Shock, trauma, despair	**Grape Hyacinth** (Pacific) for regaining balance and perspective
Birth traumas, fear of physical separation between mother and child	**Hooker's Onion** (Pacific) for feeling light-hearted and refreshed, nurturing creativity
Abuse, abandonment or psychic, emotional or physical assault	**Nootka Rose** (Pacific) for reintegrating the psyche after assault, sometimes years after the experience
Accidents and seemingly unexpected physical and emotional trauma	**Weigela** (Pacific) for integration and alignment

15
Feeling Unloved, Alienated or Abandoned

Running like a thread through these chapters, whatever the particular symptoms of unease or depression, has been the possibility of known or unknown childhood trauma. This may have occurred in our early years or even before, as negative emotions sensed from within the womb. Experiencing rejection at such a young age is perhaps the strongest and most enduring form of the loss of love but, of course, it is by no means the only one. Many children and young people grow up in uncaring environments, and suffer greatly from it. Frequently they learn hatred in return, but there are other reactions too.

Feeling alienated

Some people who didn't experience enough love in childhood feel, later, that they never had a home, or as if they come from another planet.

To children, who come from a place of love to be nurtured until they are ready to do their work in the world, not feeling wanted is the same as not being loved. Babies deal only in love; it is the one currency they know and they bring a store of it with them. Their expectation, possibly the sole expectation they are aware of on arrival, is to have that love returned. When it is not, these children simply bury their loss and forget they ever experienced it. But in fact the message is consigned to their subconscious, where it is maintained at the cost of a significant amount of vital energy. They remain confused in some way about love, particularly parental love, without really knowing why. It is comparatively rare for children to understand clearly that they were denied love in their early life, but it is possible for some to recognise this themselves.

When the message received by the child is re-experienced later in life, it can be so painful that it causes depression and poor mental health. However, the universe seems to have a feasible motive for allowing it to happen: it requires the input of its most creative creatures, humans; these creative humans can be stimulated to do their very best by looking for the love that they crave outside of the family. This is perhaps one

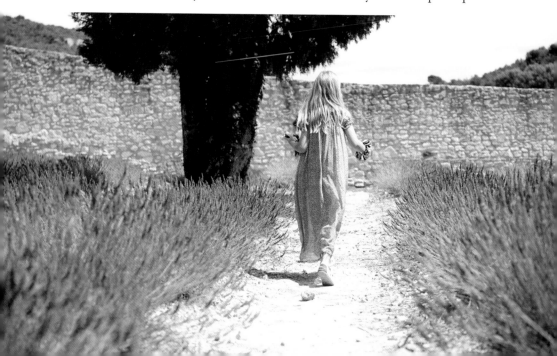

explanation of why genius has so often been seen to lie very close to madness.

How does this translate into lived experience? I think Gilda's story gives an example, albeit rather an extreme one, but it helps to illustrate the disconnectedness that can arise from childhood trauma.

Case study: Gilda
Hopelessness, feeling unwanted (psychosis)

Gilda was brought to me in an uncommunicative state, and for the first session her carer, who was a relative, had to give me Gilda's background. Following a recent episode, Gilda's anti-psychotic drug had been increased in dosage. I was given no information as to what might have triggered her latest breakdown, but her original psychotic episode had apparently occurred some years previously, following a very brief flirtation with a recreational drug.

I uncovered in her a deep sense of **loneliness** and **obstinacy**, and an even deeper feeling of **hopelessness**. I perceived that she felt she could get no help, and yet her energy (ch'i) seemed to be high. I believe that she had **felt unwanted** from the very beginning, and that she had experienced an illness between the ages of seven and fourteen. There appeared to be a significant amount of ongoing **conflict** at home even now, which Gilda found distressing.

I gave her two Wildflower essences:
- **White Archangel**, which 'helps to process anger, encourages humility and to communicate with the heart; grounding'
- **Sweet Dreams**, which 'feels like you are back in your mother's arms, comforted, nurtured and supported; encourages love'

I learned the next day that this had led to an immediate and remarkable improvement in her condition. By her second session the sense of loneliness and hopelessness had receded, and she was able to tell me that a long-term relationship had broken up recently. She said that her recent episode had taken her back to her early childhood illness, which she connected with antagonism in the home. She also linked her original breakdown to an earlier stage in the long-term relationship, when she had had an abortion.

This time I selected essences from the Bloesem Remedies range:

- **Stinkende Gouwe (Greater Celandine)**, which 'eliminates emotional poisons, getting rid of anything that you no longer need or makes you ill'
- **Living Starlight**, which 'gives relaxation and releases you from everything that is not part of your being'
- **Pepermunt**, which 'helps you digest everything which is difficult, especially what is happening in this moment in your life and in the world'

These three essences seemed to dissolve the obstinacy – the wound left by the lack of love she received from her mother and father – and more besides. Her energy remained high and steady and her psychosis had diminished. I now chose:

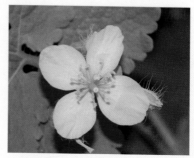

Greater Celandine

- **Devic** essence (White Light), which 'assists us to care for ourselves and others on a spiritual level and brings about a devotional, nurturing quality within us for ourselves and others'

- **Angelic** (White Light), which stimulates creativity

At her next session she reported that she was feeling scapegoated at home. I gave her:

- **Stepping Ahead Now** (Dancing Light) – 'you've done the work; now go forth into that which you have prepared'
- **Sea Turtle** (Pacific) 'for grace, grounding and transformation'

A month later, she reported that the pain of separation from her partner was now becoming much easier to manage. She was back in touch with her creativity, which for her meant sketching, sculpture and spirituality. Her anti-psychotic drug was also being steadily reduced, with no ill effect. I suggested Green Man Tree's essence **Tamarisk**, which 'is about understanding one's place at the centre of creation'. During the next few months she was able to come off the anti-psychotic drug completely.

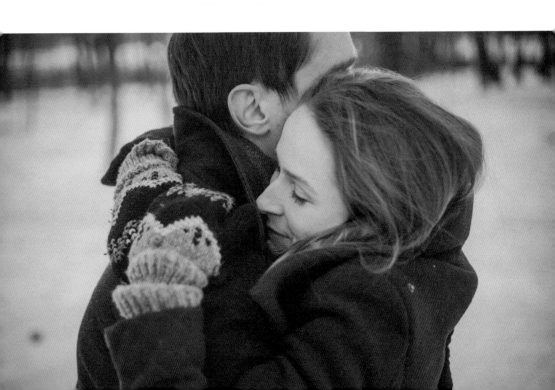

Treatment

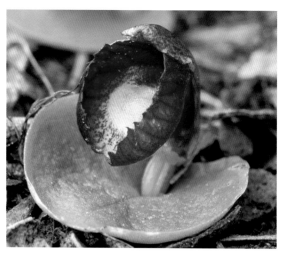

Red Helmet Orchid

Formula Leucantha from Florais de St Germain in Brazil deals very effectively with the message of **not feeling wanted** by people who matter (in or outside the family). And this is supported by **Red Helmet Orchid** from Australian Bush Flowers, an essence for dealing with **father issues**.

Habitually, these essences create a significant jump in the person's energy. If their energy drops again and feelings of being unwanted return, then the essences simply need to be repeated. But these are by no means the only essences that address the problem. Turn to page 202 to find out more about selecting and sourcing these essences.

Symptoms	Remedy
Feelings of abandonment resulting in needy or manipulative behaviour	**Chicory** (Bach) for love and care that gives freely to others
Soul feeling of profound emptiness	**Heather** (Bach) for inner tranquillity, emotional self-sufficiency
Unloved, rejected, abandoned, isolated, alienated	**Holly** (Bach) for the conquering all through love
Despair of the soul, feeling abandoned by God	**Sweet Chestnut** (Bach) for a light shining in the darkness

Symptoms	Remedy
Old learned patterns of excessively harsh self-judgement	**Bladder Senna** (Bailey) for self-compassion and self-understanding
Difficulties from our childhood experiences and conditioning	**Childhood** (Bailey) for dissolving old patterns and coming up to date
Feeling alienated and alone	**Deep Red Peony** (Bailey) for growing up as a spiritual being in a material universe
Needing to connect the heart to the love of God	**Sacred Lotus** (Bailey) for opening up to the love of the infinite and radiating that knowledge
A childhood deprived of true love, bereft and unable to love others	**Valerian** (Bailey) for the development of self-love and self-esteem
Closed, fear of lack, greed, rigidity	**Bluebell** (Bush) for opening the heart, belief in abundance, universal trust, joyful sharing
Unable to accept praise, excessive generosity	**Philotheca** (Bush) for being open to receive love and acknowledgement from others
Vague, disconnected, split, lack of focus, daydreaming	**Red Lily** (Bush) for realising you are a loving child of a loving God
Lack of loving bonds between children and parents	**Red Helmet Orchid and Bottlebrush** (Bush) for bonding, sensitivity, respect and consideration with and for fathers and mothers
Prejudice, narrow-mindedness	**Slender Rice Flower** (Bush) for humility, group harmony, co-operation, perception of beauty in others
Chasm in the heart from abandonment or alienation from others	**Tall Yellow Top** (Bush) for a sense of belonging, acceptance of self and others, knowing you are home
Feeling rejected and abandoned by your father	**Baby Blue Eyes** (FES) for feeling supported and loved, especially by men
Alienation from your sexual identity	**Calla Lily** (FES) for clarity about sexual identity, sexual self-acceptance
Feeling rejected by mother *in utero* or in early infancy	**Evening Primrose** (FES) for being able to open emotionally and form deep, committed relationships

119

Symptoms	Remedy
Feeling abandoned due to lack of bonding with the mother	**Mariposa Lily** (FES) for the ability to nurture and be nurtured
Profound alienation, not feeling at home on Earth	**Shooting Star** (FES) for cosmic consciousness warmed with caring for all that is human and earthly
Social alienation and isolation, not feeling at home	**Sweet Pea** (FES) for commitment to community, a sense of one's place on Earth
Feeling an outsider or stranger	**Violet** (FES) for being socially responsive but self-contained
Homesickness, longing, abandonment	**Arbutus** (Pacific) for being at home in the world, bonding with fathers
Coldness, uncaring, inability to feel, emotional wounds	**Fireweed** (Pacific) for realising the abundance of love within and without
Sophistication, over-control, rigidity	**Lily of the Valley** (Pacific) for simplicity, innocence, unconditional love
Weariness, abuse, abandonment	**Nootka Rose** (Pacific) for expressing love of life, laughter and joy
Anger and lack of perspective	**Pearly Everlasting** (Pacific) for commitment, devotion, service
Self-loathing	**Vanilla Leaf** (Pacific) for love of self
Not feeling wanted for whatever reason	**Formula Leucantha** (St Germain) for a sense of being nurtured

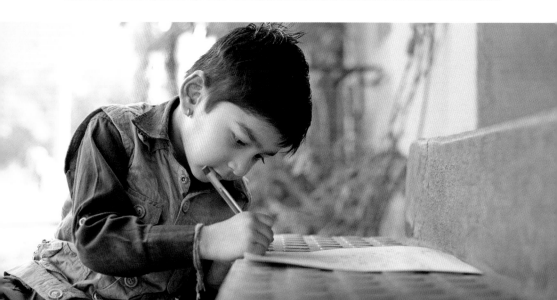

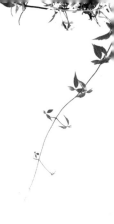

16
Family Conflict

Children are wonderfully resilient and can survive and thrive even in the most difficult circumstances. This resilience usually comes from a strong and supportive family; a platoon mentality develops where the strength of one contributes to the strength of all. However, when a parent, carer, close others, or unchecked siblings are the source of stresses and negativity, children may be unable to digest and grow through those experiences. Growth continues, as it must, but only at the expense of burying the indigestible difficulties, and only at a cost to the child's full charge of vital energy, which is perpetually depleted by the need to keep the difficult stuff suppressed.

Learning from difficult times

An atmosphere of family conflict can also be seen as a form of education in its own way. By recognising the problems we have faced, we can seek help to overcome them and grow stronger.

Angela's story illustrates not only how not feeling wanted by her father set the ground for later depression, but also how loss can trigger a depressive episode.

Case study: Angela
Depression since childhood

Angela was taken for counselling as a child and thought of herself as the black sheep of the family. She felt that her father had always undermined her self-image and she had given up speaking to him. She felt put down not only by him, but also by her male boss, and saw herself as having a **difficult, reactive personality**. She felt **despondent** and **depressed** and lacking a clear direction: 'I don't get panic attacks but **I worry**.'

I first gave her:

- ❀ **Monga Waratah** (Bush) which 'addresses the negative conditions of disempowerment; of being overly needy; ... feeling choked or stifled in situations or relationships and feeling not able or strong enough to leave'

- ❀ **Komkommerkruid** (**Borage**) (Bloesem Remedies) 'for handling things from the heart rather than the head'

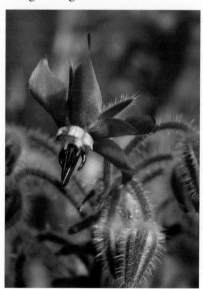

A month later she was feeling trapped and unable to relax; she had physical trouble with haemorrhoids; but her emotional health was improving – she was communicating with her father again, and her vital energy had increased significantly. I then gave:

Borage

- ❁ **Paarse Dovenetel (Red Henbit)** (Bloesem) 'for flushing away confrontational situations ... and for not being able to grow and be who we really are'
- ❁ **Vital Balance** combination (Fox Mountain) 'for clearing away blocks that prevent healing'

At the next session she was looking better following a month's holiday with her boyfriend. Her haemorrhoids had retreated and she seemed to be getting more out of her job. Her energy had increased again, but her relationship with her father had not necessarily improved. Four essences came to mind:

- ❁ **Goatsbeard** (Pacific) which 'enables us to see ourselves as calm and relaxed in stressful situations'
- ❁ **Black-Eyed Susan** (Fox Mountain) for 'frustration, bitterness, irritability'
- ❁ **Horseradish** (Fox Mountain) for those 'who are having trouble moving beyond the past reality of pain; brings the ability to accept that the past has been bitter and that now it is time to move on and create more nourishing realities'

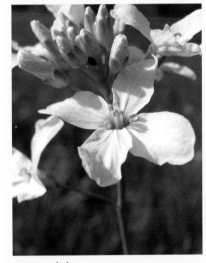

Horseradish

- ❁ **Vision Quest** (Fox Mountain) to stimulate her creativity

She did well for some time, but many months later she was feeling battered by life and the possibility of losing her job. Her vital energy had dropped, and suggested a need for self-nurture.

She took:

- **Tibetan Rock Rose** (PHI), which 'enables us to accept and love ourselves as we are'
- **Lammas** (Corryn Webb) to align with the rhythms of the Earth

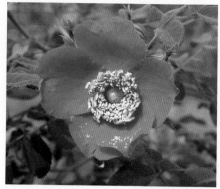

Tibetan Rock Rose

At a later session she had sadly lost her job and was taking a bleak view of her prospects. It was very clear that she was suffering from depression and her energy had dropped to an all-time low. I gave her:

- **Fire** (White Light), of which Ian White writes, 'There is no middle ground with this essence. There is nowhere to go except forward'
- **Salamander** (Wild Earth) 'for those who are going through a process of deep emotional healing'

When these essences had done their work her energy had improved substantially and she was ready for life's new challenges.

Treatment

As you read the suggested essences in the following table, you may feel unsure of who should be taking the essence from the brief description provided. Mother or son? Father or daughter? In fact, the symptoms could apply to either. But remember that this is a family affair, not confined to one generation. The problem may have been going on over several generations. The important thing is to take the essence that you feel may shift things. If you are in doubt, take it yourself and perhaps clarification will come or,

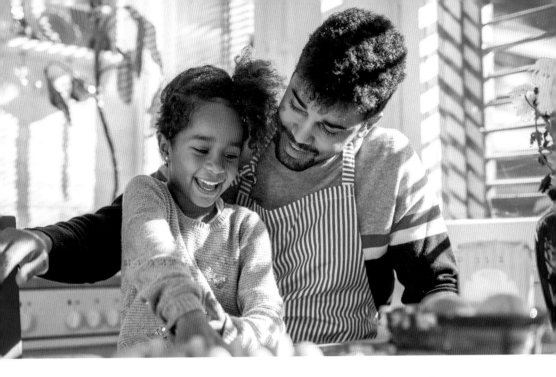

better still, forgiveness, and a new way of looking at things. Turn to page 202 to find out more about selecting and sourcing these essences.

Symptoms	Remedy
Overly critical of your child	**Beech** (Bach) for tolerance, seeing the good within each person, ability to praise others
Feelings of abandonment resulting in needy or manipulative behaviour	**Chicory** (Bach) for love and care that gives freely to others
Soul feeling of profound emptiness	**Heather** (Bach) for inner tranquillity, emotional self-sufficiency
Unloved, rejected, abandoned, isolated, alienated	**Holly** (Bach) for conquering all through love
Internalising guilt due to harsh or strict parenting	**Pine** (Bach) for self-acceptance, freedom to move forward despite past mistakes
Exerting harsh or extreme control over children	**Vine** (Bach) for recognition of the individuality of others

Symptoms	Remedy
The subservient child, dominated by others	**Bracken** (Bailey) for making our own assessments and taking responsibility
Adult life feels threatening	**Charlock** (Bailey) for being a competent, confident, joyful adult
Difficulties from our childhood experiences and conditioning	**Childhood** (Bailey) for dissolving old patterns and coming up to date
Deprived of true love in childhood	**Valerian** (Bailey) for the development of self-love
Conflict over sharing with rest of family	**Bluebell** (Bush) for belief in abundance, joyful sharing
Enmeshed in negative family patterns, for recipients of abuse and prejudice	**Boab** (Bush) for personal freedom by releasing family patterns
Feuding between mother and children	**Bottlebrush** (Bush) for serenity and calm, ability to cope and move on
Resentment and bitterness towards close family	**Dagger Hakea** (Bush) for forgiveness and open expression of feelings
Family prejudices that have been taught rather than experienced	**Freshwater Mangrove** (Bush) for healthy questioning of traditional standards and beliefs
Family conflict arising based on early childhood jealousy	**Mountain Devil** (Bush) for unconditional love, healthy boundaries, forgiveness
Feuding between father and children	**Red Helmet Orchid** (Bush) for male bonding, sensitivity, respect, consideration
Disturbed relationship with father often involving abuse or abandonment	**Baby Blue Eyes** (FES) for feeling supported and loved, especially by men
Hysterical parenting tendencies creating 'trauma-drama' family situations	**Canyon Dudleya** (FES) for an ordered and simple approach to parenting and homemaking
Vacillating between being over strict or overly permissive as a parent	**Quince** (FES) for loving strength and firm loving
Conflict with or abuse from father or other male family members	**Saguaro** (FES) for healing relationship with elders or male family members

Symptoms	Remedy
Episodes of rage or power battles with your child	**Scarlet Monkeyflower** (FES) for direct and clear communication of deep feelings
Vacillating sense of Self, inflation or self-effacement, low self-esteem or arrogance owing to poor relationship with father	**Sunflower** (FES) for general healing of relationship with father and self-image internalised from the father
Parenting as a grim responsibility, lack of joy or spontaneity in parenting	**Zinnia** (FES) for playing with and enjoying your child's world, contacting your own inner child
Family power struggle	**Alum Root** (Pacific) for grace, trust, light-heartedness
Family (and other) conflict	**Narcissus** (Pacific) for identification and resolution of conflict by going to the centre of the problem or fear
Lack of perspective, anger	**Pearly Everlasting** (Pacific) for commitment to relationship, devotion
Grudges, resentment, judgemental	**Salal** (Pacific) for forgiveness

17
Negative Programming Learned in Childhood

As with computers, children can be programmed in a certain way. Much of our learning comes from being programmed by parents, carers, teachers or peers. Ideally, this programming is more or less beneficial, a preparation for life, and for fitting in with society. But it can be harmful if our parents or carers expose us to unhelpful or antisocial ideas that we begin to take on as 'normal'. It is for this sad reason that some sufferers of physical or sexual abuse can, when they have their own children, continue the cycle.

In fact, children seem to have an innate programming of their own, which is geared to high expectations, but this 'good' or 'normal' programming can still be overcome by constant, and often painful, repetition of negative influences. If children are continually led into believing that bad, painful and negative behaviours are the norm, they bury the experiences so they can focus on their primary form of programming: that of development and growth, coded into us by nature. However, maintaining the suppression of negative experiences in our subconscious uses up vital energy.

Teenage depression and 'bad behaviour'

At times of transition in our lives, such as puberty, when all our energy is required for development, the energy usually used to suppress negative programming is diverted, and material can burst from the subconscious in ways which are categorised as 'bad behaviour' or mental disorders of some kind.

Besides abuse, other forms of negative programming can arise from:
- parental conflict and breakup
- parental constraint
- neglect
- insecurity
- perception of failure

Sometimes the programming we internalised is buried, sometimes it is worn for all to see, subject to our societal constraints. One of the common characteristics is that it becomes harder and harder to recognise the damage in childhood we have received, which inevitably poses difficulties in later life. Our egos, as they grow, develop a layer of protection. The greater the difficulties to which we have been exposed growing up, the stronger our walls of protection tend to become.

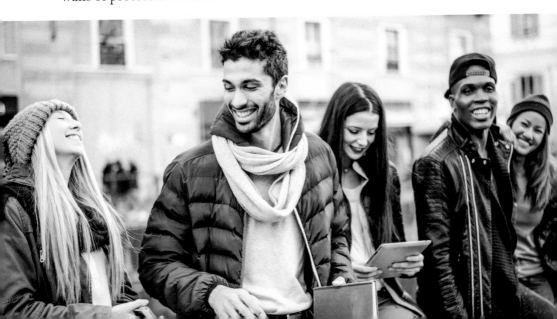

Treatment

The task of flower essences here is to gently dissolve the old programming and allow us to rediscover ourselves, so that our interrupted or distorted development can be continued along more positive lines, and with greater vital energy.

Finding your path in life

Everyone arrives on Earth with a range of potential paths they can choose to follow. If children are treated harshly by their carers, their free will is eroded and they can struggle to follow any path until help arrives, usually in the form of therapy of some kind.

It can be very difficult for us to reset our programming on our own – we are much more complex than computers. Here are some of the essences which help. You may also find Chapter 16 on Family Conflict helpful. Turn to page 202 to find out more about selecting and sourcing these essences.

Symptoms	Remedy
Seeing others critically, harsh judgement	**Beech** (Bach) for tolerance, seeing the good within each person, ability to praise others
Yearning for positive things from the past	**Heather** (Bach) for unblocking suppressed qualities and restrictions
Inability to open heart to love for others	**Holly** (Bach) for heartfelt compassion, ability to express gratitude to others
Trying to repress the free will of others	**Vine** (Bach) for recognition of others' individuality
Bitter and resentful, unable to forgive	**Willow** (Bach) for acceptance, taking responsibility for your situation in life

Symptoms	Remedy
The subservient child, dominated by others	**Bracken** (Bailey) for making your own assessments and taking responsibility
Deeply entrenched behavioural patterns that dominate our lives	**Cellular Memory combination** (Bailey) for lifting these blocks
Difficulties from our childhood experiences and conditioning	**Childhood combination** (Bailey) for dissolving old patterns and coming up to date
Old habits that are holding us back	**Giant Bellflower** (Bailey) for changing your life
A narrow view of the world and ourselves	**Pink Purslane** (Bailey) for leaving past attitudes behind and embracing empowerment
Repressed energies	**Round-headed Leek** (Bailey) for resolving old, deeply hidden hurts
Blocked off energies and memories of the distant past	**Wood Anemone** (Bailey) for regaining your lost powers
Overly self-critical	**Five Corners** (Bush) for love and acceptance of self
Judgemental because of learnt prejudice	**Freshwater Mangrove** (Bush) for openness to new experiences, perceptions and people
Cynical and suspicious attitude to life and other people	**Mountain Devil** (Bush) for unconditional love, forgiveness
Old deep hurt and pain from traumatic abuse	**Pink Mulla Mulla** (Bush) for deep spiritual healing, trusting and opening up
Expecting the worst of life because of past experience	**Sunshine Wattle** (Bush) for optimism, acceptance of beauty and joy in the present
Dark depression after abuse	**Waratah** (Bush) for courage to move on
Judgemental	**Yellow Cowslip Orchid** (Bush) for impartiality, stepping back from emotions
Lack of awareness of your 'shadow' self	**Black-Eyed Susan** (FES) for penetrating insight and self-aware behaviour
Toxicity due to violence, post-traumatic stress or drugs	**Chapparal** (FES) for balanced psychic awareness

131

Symptoms	Remedy
Repression of emotions and sexual feelings due to emotional and sexual abuse in childhood, fear of parenthood	**Evening Primrose** (FES) for awareness and healing of painful early emotions absorbed from parents
Repression of painful childhood memories	**Golden Eardrops** (FES) for remembering and understanding experiences that define emotional history
Fear of exposure and rejection due to prior abuse and trauma	**Pink Monkeyflower** (FES) for courage to take emotional risks with others
Projection of negativity onto others, paranoia	**Oregon Grape** (FES) for loving inclusion of others, ability to trust
Vulnerable to negative influences, especially of a mental or psychic nature	**Yarrow** (FES) for compassionate and inclusive sensitivity
Addiction to toxic mental, emotional and physical patterns	**Forsythia** (Pacific) for motivation and transformation
Letting go of dysfunctional behaviour patterns	**Fuchsia** (Pacific) for peeling the layers of programming, balance
Letting go of limiting beliefs and attitudes, fear of being judged by others	**Grass Widow** (Pacific) for freedom to hold your own beliefs
Thoughts of limitation	**Hooker's Onion** (Pacific) for creative expression
Weariness following abuse or abandonment	**Nootka Rose** (Pacific) for expressing love of life, laughter and joy
Poisonous thoughts and attitudes, resentment	**Plantain** (Pacific) for releasing mental blocks and negativity

18
Mourning and Grief

We develop extremely strong bonds with our parents, children, siblings and friends – we love them and they are part of us. They become as vital as our limbs and organs, and something more besides. We 'internalise good objects' as psychotherapists say and we feel terrible pain when we lose them. This is the pain of mourning.

I think it is worth noting that mourning and depression are sometimes hard to differentiate – something Freud observed – and yet linking the two can help us to understand both processes. One is caused by the actual loss of a person, and the other by a perception of loss.[1] Mourning is not a symptom of depression but a natural process in itself. Of course we are inconsolably sad when someone we love dies, and it is important for us to go through these emotions to acknowledge the effect that person had on our lives and on the world.

Flower essences can help with grief

The impact felt by loss can trigger something similar to depression and cause many symptoms that can be helped by flower essences.

Apart from the sense of loss, some other difficult emotions are bound up with mourning, which can be defined in **the five stages of grief: denial, anger, bargaining, depression and acceptance.**[2] As I said in Chapter 9 on Anger, love always seems to lie beneath our painful emotions. We are angry because someone we love has hurt us; we feel a sense of loss because someone we love has gone.

The pain of grief

The pain of grief is just as much a part of life as the joy of love. It is, perhaps, the price we pay for love, the cost of commitment. To ignore this fact, or to pretend that it is not so, is to put on emotional blinkers, which leaves us unprepared for the losses that will inevitably occur in our lives and unprepared to help others with the losses in theirs.[3]

Parkes and Prigerson

Mourning can be very intense. I recall seeing C. S. Lewis on television, six months after the death of his wife, with tears spurting from his eyes at the memory. This kind of expression of mourning can be cathartic. Shortly afterwards, Lewis's tears – which had been almost continuous since his wife's death – stopped quite suddenly.

Express your grief

It is an important part of normal and healthy mourning to express our grief – we feel strong grief, we express strong grief, and then we can begin to move on with life.

However, sometimes we feel social pressure not to express our grief strongly and openly, and we can internalise this pressure. Then our response to pain, even great pain, can be to conceal it. Often we are trained to stoicism from an early age and if, because of this or for any other reason, we cannot mourn and move on, mourning can affect us physically. I feel sure this was the case with Manuela, who moved rapidly onward and upward when her grief over difficulties with her father were addressed.

Case study: Manuela
Unexpressed grief

Manuela, 46, came to see me suffering from pleurisy and pain under the diaphragm. She felt that she was caught in a regime of taking too many pharmaceutical drugs, which included steroids for her asthma that were being prescribed in increasingly strong doses. This asthma had first started when she went away to school for the first time aged around ten years old, but they had recently intensified. Her husband worked overseas for long periods of time and she felt **alone**, **frightened** and terribly depressed at these times. In the past she had tried to commit suicide and she did not want to feel that way again. I discovered that she had always had a very **difficult relationship with her father** who she found fierce and tyrannical, and had rebelled strongly against him.

The lungs are the seat of grief in traditional Chinese medicine and, in this peri-menopausal period, it seemed likely to me that the pleurisy indicated that she was now grappling with problems from long ago, specifically **mourning** the sense of the loss of a 'good' father, one she could look up to and trust. I selected **Sturt Desert Pea** (Bush) for dealing with grief and pain from far back in time.

A few weeks later, at her second session, the pleurisy had cleared up. She said she felt well, but **fragile**, and that she wanted to feel more confident in her new-found health. Gradually her drugs were being reduced, but she was now feeling **nervous** about re-entering life and taking on work again. I gave her:

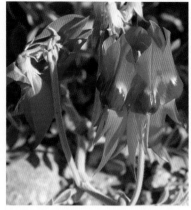

Sturt Desert Pea

- **Boerenwormkruid (Tansy)** (Bloesem Remedies) for 'when someone is always in doubt and cannot make decisions'
- **Gymea Lily** (Bush) for humility and reaching great heights – pursuing your passion

At her next visit I asked what had changed. 'I can drink!' she said. 'I've been riding my bike. I feel much better!' For a clear message now of turning inwards and being still I gave her:

- **Black-Eyed Susan** (Fox Mountain)
- **Impatiens** (Bach)

Mourning our Parents

Mourning can be particularly difficult when we grieve for the death of parents or early caregivers whose love or support was not quite satisfactory. If we are comfortable with how our parents raised us, and were more or less at peace with them when they died, it seems to me that we mourn them in the 'normal' way. There is pain. It takes a while as with any loss, and at last there is acceptance. We are left with memories.

But it certainly isn't always like that. If damage occurred during the early years, and by damage I mean wounds that endured in the psyche, such as neglect, abuse or insecurity, then there can be serious and painful work to be done. It's not uncommon for friends who know us well to comment, 'Why is she making such a fuss about his passing? She didn't even like him.'

When we experience psychological wounds in the early years, a part of us is left behind and fails to develop healthily. The death of a parent can bring that undeveloped part to the surface for re-examination and re-evaluation. We are called to come to terms with the early difficulty, and of course this is even more challenging because the old, painful feelings come back to us at the very time we are mourning the person we loved and depended on as a child.

Hopefully by then we will have learned enough through life to be able to deal with the challenge, and we can begin to grow again. Sometimes, however, the long-buried pain which surfaces is so great that we may unconsciously feel the need to bury it again, preventing us from moving on from the powerful sense of loss we feel.[4]

I believe that we need to make allowances for each individual mourning process that occurs when we lose someone close to us. The expectation among practioners of conventional medicine seems to be that 'normal mourning' lasts about one year.[5] But each person's experience is different.

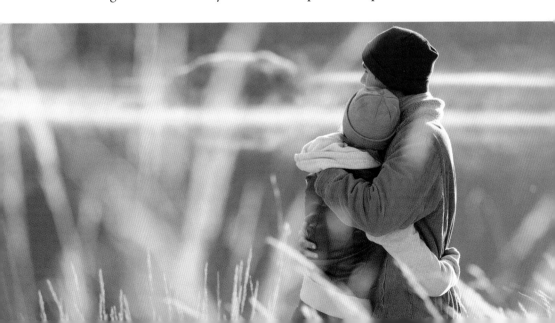

We must allow time for mourning

People have very different patterns of mourning: some take longer than others to feel better; some feel fine in the short term but are struck by mourning after several months or sometimes years, particularly on anniversaries.

This is often the case when people are shocked in the aftermath of death: they start to feel grief when they are ready; to feel so much straightaway is too much to manage. And if the mourner becomes stuck and unable to move through trauma from their past, then mourning can take even longer. In these cases the flower essences aren't just serving to help us weather a difficult year, but to take on other more complex processes over a much longer period of time.

Case study: Chris
Delayed mourning

While I was working on this section of the book I had to visit the dentist for some fillings and, following the second session and the anaesthetic that went with it, I caught a severe cold. At first I concentrated on clearing my system of the anaesthetic using Bach's **Crab Apple**. A little later, with the cold still there, I switched to remedies for keeping sinusitis at bay: Australian Bush Flowers' **Bush Iris**, **Dagger Hakea** and **Fringed Violet**. But as the days stretched into weeks and my energy remained low, and the cold had to be reconsidered as bronchitis, I realised that I was actually in mourning for the deaths of two people – my mother and my first wife – and this was preventing me from overcoming the illness.

For one reason or another I had not done the essential grieving work at the time of either of their deaths, and now it was

138

being brought home to me: my mourning was not disordered, but very much delayed. Now I looked again at the remedy I needed and this was **Sneeuwklokje (Snowdrop)** from Bloesem Remedies Nederland. Bram Zaalberg tells us that **Sneeuwklokje** 'releases deep pain, tears and old trauma that have been stored up for a long time: it brings

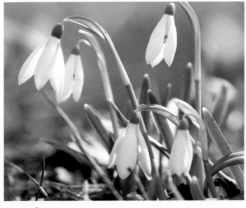

Snowdrop

a stronger trust, deep down in the depths of one's being, and is joyful and refreshing after the long, dark emotional winter'.[6] Here at least there is some differentiation: a cold or bronchitis is not the same as depression, but sometimes physical ill-health can be an indicator of deeper emotional issues that need addressing, to avoid depression setting in.

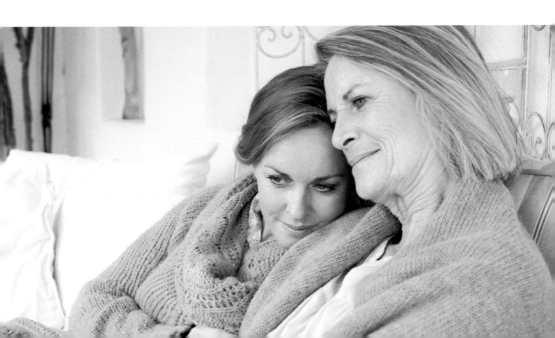

Treatment

Flower essences support the whole person – emotionally, mentally and physically – and can therefore be very helpful in alleviating a wide range of difficulties that accompany grief. When we are mourning, we often encounter problems that we may not immediately connect with grief, but which have come about as a result of our loss. Flower essences can help us to work through the layers of our grief and find the energy to move on with life. There are a number of remedies available to specifically address a spectrum of grief-related conditions, and some more general flower essences have a grief component. Turn to page 202 to find out more about selecting and sourcing these essences.

Symptoms	Remedy
Extreme pain or shock in situations of death and dying	**Five Flowers (Rescue Remedy)** (Bach) for calming, restoring peace and emotional balance
Inability to open heart to love for others	**Holly** (Bach) for bringing calm and acceptance to the heart
Feeling stuck in the past	**Honeysuckle** (Bach) for letting go so that life can go on after death
Shock following death	**Star of Bethlehem** (Bach) for soothing and calming
Feeling unable to accept the loss of a loved one	**Walnut** (Bach) for allowing transition, breaking links
Withdrawal or numbing due to grief	**Wild Rose** (Bach) for accepting the tragic events of life
Bitterness and resentment towards family	**Willow** (Bach) for acceptance, forgiveness, taking responsibility for your life situation
Bereavement or grief that is locked within us	**Grief Composite** (Bailey) for expressing grief

Symptoms	Remedy
Feeling totally bereft and others seem distant	**Dog Rose** (Bailey) for expressing grief
Resentment caused by feeling 'Why did this happen to me?'	**Sheep's Sorrel** (Bailey) for leaving bitterness behind
Emotional tension and desperation that are often part of the grieving process	**Trailing St John's Wort** (Bailey) for taking the sting out of the situation
For being 'knocked sideways' by grief	**Yin/Yang Balancer** (Bailey) for restoring balance, including physical balance
Anguish of grief	**Yorkshire Fog** (Bailey) for shedding tears to wash the grief away
Holding on to grief	**Bottlebrush** (Bush) for accepting inevitable changes
Anger at the loss of a loved one	**Dagger Hakea** (Bush) for open expression of feelings
Grief in a child after death or separation from a parent	**Little Flannel Flower** (Bush) for being carefree, playful and joyful
Deep hurt, even going back to an earlier incarnation	**Pink Mulla Mulla** (Bush) for spiritual healing, trusting and opening up
Raw emotions associated with death of a loved one	**Red Suva Frangipani** (Bush) for feeling calm and nurtured, inner peace and strength to cope
Deep hurt going back a long time	**Sturt Desert Pea** (Bush) for releasing deep-held grief and sadness
Guilt associated with loss	**Sturt Desert Rose** (Bush) for courage, conviction, being true to self
Entangled in relationships based on fear, possessiveness or neediness	**Bleeding Heart** (FES) for emotional freedom to love others unconditionally
Heavy-heartedness or grief	**Borage** (FES) for buoyant courage and optimism
Grief or emotional pain stuck in the body	**Dandelion** (FES) for dynamic physical energy and expressive life force

141

Symptoms	Remedy
Holding on to deeply-seated pain or grief	**Fuchsia** (FES) for the ability to express intense feelings
Feelings of pain, grief and trauma from childhood	**Golden Ear Drops** (FES) for remembering and understanding experiences that define emotional history
Need to release dysfunctional aspects within the personality	**Sagebrush** (FES) for accepting the pain and emptiness of any kind of loss
Deeply internalised pain stored in the heart and chest	**Yerba Santa** (FES) for capacity to express a full range of emotions, especially pain and sadness
Loss and anger	**Orange Honeysuckle** (Pacific) for evoking peaceful creativity
Grief, deep sadness	**Purple Crocus** (Pacific) for resolving tension generated from grief and loss

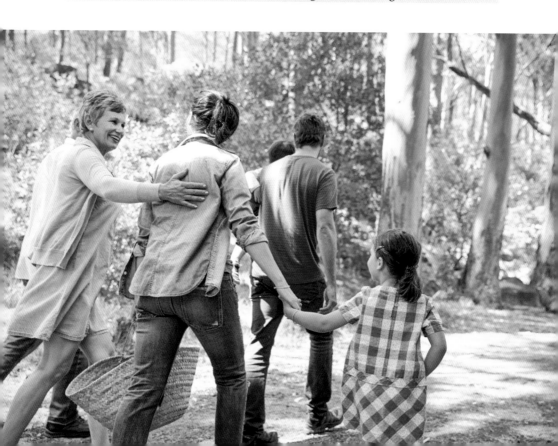

19
Loss

What is loss?

Anything that we love – in which we have 'invested' – becomes part of us and we feel its loss painfully. We mourn that loss, whether it is the loss of a person or not.

Depression is often connected to an earlier loss, and essentially there is very little difference between loss and grief. What has been lost is love; if the person (expectation, dream, or object) in whom our love was invested goes, then our love goes with them. First, perhaps, we experience a period of denial, followed by anger and outrage: all typical accompaniments to the process of grief (see Chapter 18).

I believe that we all come from a spiritual place where love is the currency. When we arrive in the physical world, ideally protected by a loving family, we grow and, bit by bit, we learn about the other currencies of the physical world, such as money, power and conflict at a rate we can assimilate. We develop into complex emotional adults who can cope with and contribute to our constantly changing universe. That, at least, is the situation in 'normal' development. If our development is interrupted by loss in early life, our understanding of the world as a place where love is, usually located in our parents, can be forcibly and dramatically changed. Love can turn within a matter of days to anger, outrage and then to hatred. If this happens in childhood, the sense of loss can be so great that it leaves an indelible wound in the psyche, and children can even lose their sense of refuge or home. As a result of this some people reach adulthood without an idea of a true, safe home.

How loss and trauma affect children

My favourite philosopher/psychologist, Ken Wilber, describes what happens when childhood development is interrupted by trauma between the ages of three and nine (the egocentric stage). The damaged aspect of the self splits off, but the rest continues its development ('It might bleed all over the place, but it keeps climbing'), leaving the damaged aspect behind, with its development capability impaired, continuing to interpret the world through the senses of a young child. The internal conflict between the stuck part and the developed part 'can be devastating. This is not an external conflict; it is a civil war'. [1]

When a loss occurs in later life, the pain can be very intense as it reawakens an earlier trauma, an invisible wound, which has not been fully healed. If the loss reawakens the inexpressible anger we felt after the original loss, not expressing it can be particularly exhausting and the depression particularly pervasive, because anger is such a powerful force.

Loss isn't only a response to death

We experience loss in response to a wide range of different situations. The key, always, is the degree of love invested in a person or an activity. We may invest our love in a totally unsuitable partner, in a job, in retirement, in a cherished dream, or in the lost chance of being a child.

Case study: Esther
Childhood abuse,
self-destructive behaviour

Esther was the youngest in her family by several years and had **not been wanted** by her parents. Her young life had been lonely, and she had experienced both **physical and sexual abuse**. As a result, she had become very **self-destructive** as an adult, involving herself in **drink, drugs** and **obsessive overworking**. She came to see me at the time of a career change, suffering from very **low self-esteem**, depressed, pushing away those closest to her by her abrasive behaviour, testing her new relationship to the limits, and sleeping badly. Her parents had died in quick succession shortly after her previous relationship had ended. Now she had given up her earlier excesses and was looking for emotional wellbeing. She felt loved, capable, secure in her home, perhaps for the first time – and yet she still felt **hopeless**.

The first remedy I gave her was Bach's **Rock Rose** for bred-in-the-bone fear, and she felt a subtle but significant change, which improved her feelings towards her closest connections. From her second session she took away **Wild Rose**:

'A baby that has been crying for its mother for hours will at some point give up hope of its mother ever coming to relieve its hunger. Feeling utterly deserted and in complete emptiness it becomes resigned to its fate.'[2]

Afterwards Esther reported feeling moments of happiness, and the heaviness having been lifted from her shoulders. Her self-esteem had improved and her expectations of work changed for the better.

Nonetheless she needed a third remedy for desperation: Bach's **Sweet Chestnut** helps

'...when the anguish is so great as to seem to be unbearable. When the mind or body feels as if it had borne to the uttermost limit of its endurance, and that now it must give way.'[3]

During the next few months she reconnected with an aunt and other family members with whom she had lost touch, and managed a very intense project at work. Her energy had improved considerably.

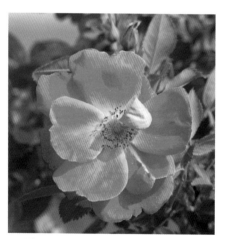

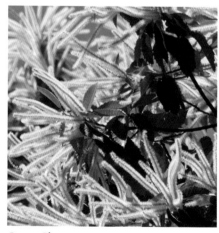

Wild Rose

Sweet Chestnut

When we have sustained an unhealed wound from an early loss too great for us to deal with at the time, such as Esther's experience of abuse, we can find ourselves pitched back into that early painful place, even when we are feeling comparatively secure. The new, seemingly smaller loss 'codes' for the early, original large loss and we are given another opportunity to deal with unfinished business.

There really does appear to be a point to all this discomfort. The human race is very creative, but the fruits of this creativity are not achieved by sitting comfortably. When the protection provided by the love and support of family and friends is stripped away from us, we have to turn to our own resources, and we discover that our most enduring source of love and support comes from within ourselves.

Being creative is therapeutic

When we are doing something worthwhile for the benefit of the universe, depression and the pain of loss tend to lose their strong hold over us. But when our creative drive pauses, or a project ends, the challenges that have defeated us in the past can reappear.

If we isolate the trigger that tipped us into depression and trace it to its roots, we can reunite the repressed, damaged aspects of our psyche with the love which has always been within us. Then we can bring love to the surface, both for our own benefit and to be shared with others.

Treatment

Each person's loss is uniquely different and will require different remedies. Have a look through the other chapter titles in Part Two of this book to see if any resonate with you. The essences outlined for grieving, Chapter 18 may be helpful, as well as the following ones, which are particularly adapted to loss:

Grieving (Fox Mountain)

'It addresses all types of loss, **loss from death**, the **loss of a relationship**, the **loss of a dream**, and the **lost chance to be a child** due to a **dysfunctional family life** ... This essence has been helping people release their whole lifetime reservoir of grief and yet it seems to release it painlessly, keeping the ego out of the process.'[4]

Angelica (FES)

Helps us feel 'protection and guidance from spiritual beings, especially at threshold experiences such as **birth and death**'.

Bleeding Heart (FES)

For those who 'suffer enormous pain and **broken-heartedness** because their feelings have been poured out so completely into another soul who is no longer present. Perhaps this happens because a loved one has died, or a cherished friend or family member has moved away. Most frequently, such anguish arises in personal relationships which have dissolved'.

Love-Lies-Bleeding (FES)

To initiate 'transcendent consciousness, the ability to **move beyond personal pain**, suffering or mental anguish by finding larger, transpersonal meaning in such suffering'.

Rock Rose (Bach)

For some people, loss stimulates **fear** (for example when the death of others reminds us of our own mortality) and Dr Bach often prescribed **Rock Rose** for very great fear.

Wild Rose (Bach)

A sense of **helplessness** can be part of loss, and **Wild Rose** is a good remedy for this.

Sweet Chestnut (Bach)

For people who feel **desperate**, sometimes in relation to loss: 'when there is nothing but destruction and annihilation left to face.'

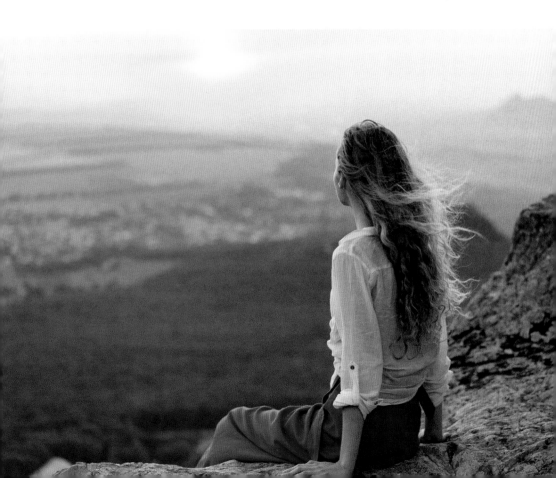

20
Emotional and Physical Abuse

Emotional and physical abuse cause deep psychological wounds, the intensity of which can lead us to become very ill. If you have suffered abuse it's important to talk to someone and seek medical help – a wide range of therapies are available, which can make a huge difference to your wellbeing.

The terrible truth in many cases of abuse, both throughout history and more recently (for example, institutional child abuse) is that abusive trauma has been repeatedly rediscovered, diagnosed with great accuracy, and then swept under the carpet because the true cause was simply not socially acceptable.[1] Two examples of this:

- ❀ **'Hysteria'**, which Freud and others demonstrated to be directly attributable to the sexual abuse of women in the 1890s.
- ❀ **PTSD** (post-traumatic stress disorder) or **shellshock**, which causes soldiers to suffer headaches and flashbacks so intense that they are unable to sustain normal working life. PTSD has only become a recognised condition relatively recently.

There are political reasons for this institutional amnesia, but that should not make such abhorrent abuse of power acceptable. Sometimes the family institution mirrors this amnesia and itself denies the existence of abuse – for example, rape and incest are denied by families to preserve their reputation.

We forget what really happened

One of the key aspects of psychological trauma resulting from abuse is amnesia and confusion over the event itself.

The process of repressing a seriously traumatic experience is a form of amnesia. A client once presented herself to me for treatment implying rather than stating that she had been sexually abused by her father. She wasn't sure, but she thought this may have occurred. There were several remedies that I thought might help boost her energy without having to resolve the matter one way or another and she went away with these. By the next time I saw her, she had become completely clear that she *had* been abused by her father and, furthermore, her sister had been able to confirm this.

Children blame themselves

Young children are egocentric: they believe the world revolves around them. An outcome of this is that they may take responsibility for events, sometimes awful or tragic ones, that they are clearly not responsible for.

When psychologist Arnhild Lauveng was three years old her father was diagnosed with cancer. When she was five he died. Lauveng believed that her father's death occurred through her own failure, and a dreadful event became even more dreadful. So dreadful, in fact, that she buried the event and its associated feelings in her subconscious, sacrificing a great deal of her vital energy in the process. And, as is the way of children who detect a hidden weakness in another, she was picked on unmercifully at school. So her life was always less than happy and, by the age of seventeen, she started to hear voices, and then things went from bad to worse...

> The Captain and the other voices constantly screamed in my head and said I was a bad person; I was always hungry and tired, because The Captain wouldn't let me sleep or eat enough, and he said he would kill me if I did not obey. Even at that time I knew he would use my body to kill me, my arms would get the rope or my legs would jump out of the window.[2]
>
> *Arnhild Lauveng*

We can see, in her story, that the appearance of 'The Captain' – an internalised figure that punishes her – makes sense in her situation. Healing the core issue, which in Lauveng's case was the belief that she was to blame for her father's death and the shocking loss of him and his love, went on to prove very helpful in treating her, and she was able to recover from her illness.

Listening to *your* story

Flower essence therapists 'look for the unique' in mental illness, we listen to each person's story and then treat the core issue rather than the psychosis.

152

Treatment

In addition to flower essences, it's important to seek further medical advice if you have suffered abuse. Other supportive measures can be taken, for example, my client, Mortimer, told me that his nightmares stopped once he stopped seeing his family.

One essence which comes up again and again for my patients in the context of traumatic backgrounds is:

Splendid Mariposa (Butterfly) Lily (FES)

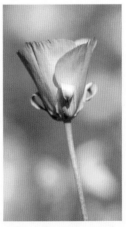

Patterns of imbalance: orphan state of consciousness as a root condition of humanity; soul pain and feelings of abandonment due to world trauma and warfare; divisions in the human family due to race, religion, nation, class, ecological disaster or warfare.

Positive qualities: soul alignment with the Mother of the World; capacity to recognise all members of the human race as having one Mother; ability to activate transcendent forces of mothering and mercy for all of the human family.

Splendid Mariposa Lily

The following are some of the issues that may arise, in no particular order, as a result of severe abuse. In addition, a fuller range of essences dealing with these and other related issues can be found in the Treatment sections of the earlier chapters – look through the chapter titles to sense which resonate with you. Turn to page 202 to find out more about selecting and sourcing these essences.

Shock

Symptoms	Remedy
Extreme pain or shock in a wide range of situations	**Five Flowers (Rescue Remedy)** (Bach) for calming, restoring peace and emotional balance
Shock or trauma, either recent or past	**Star of Bethlehem** (Bach) for soothing and calming, sense of wholeness
Damage to aura, distress	**Fringed Violet** (Bush) for healing the aura damaged by trauma

Loss of the mother

Symptoms	Remedy
Loss of the mother, a sense that love is not understood	**Formula Leucantha** (Florais de St Germain) for reconnection with and understanding of love and mothering
Feelings of childhood abandonment and abuse, orphan state of consciousness	**Splendid Mariposa Lily** (FES) for acceptance to the heart
Resentment, bitterness towards anyone close	**Dagger Hakea** (Bush) for forgiveness, open expression of feeling
Repressed anger which needs to be brought to awareness	**Black-Eyed Susan** (FES) for penetrating insight and self-aware behaviour

Encouraging creativity

Symptoms	Remedy
For indecisive, scattered people, underachievers	**Wild Oat** (Bach) for showing us how we can serve, by finding our true vocation or calling
Loss of identity or direction, anger	**Orange Honeysuckle** (Pacific) for inner direction, creative expression

154

Transition

Symptoms	Remedy
Needing to move through a developmental stage	**Walnut** (Bach) for allowing transition, breaking links
As above	**Transition Essence** (Bailey) for the past making way for the new
As above	**Transition Essence** (Bush) for forging a clear path on which to move forward

Stabilisation

Symptoms	Remedy
Instability following intense personal change	**Royal Highness** (Perelandra) for stabilising after change and development

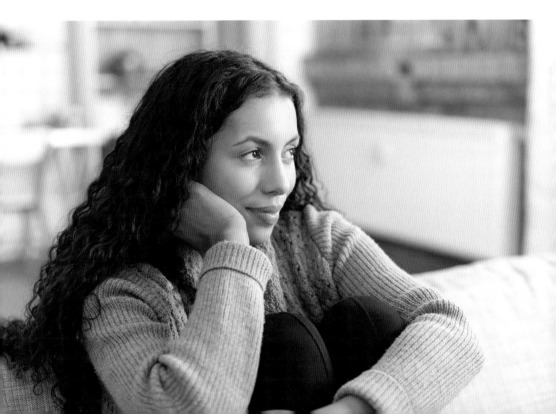

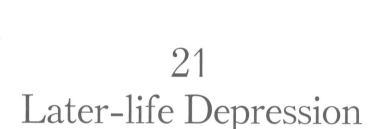

21
Later-life Depression

Many issues can lie at the core of late-onset depression: persistent failing health of one kind or another, or existential concerns about the meaning of life after retirement in the midst of our largely youth-oriented culture. Sometimes milestone birthdays prompt a re-evaluation of life and its meaning, and as a result, partnerships that have been stable for years can start to crack.

Retirement can trigger depression

People can frequently be nudged into a state of depression by a sense of loss if they have identified very closely with their jobs. (See Chapter 19 for advice on loss)

Difficulties in life that have not been satisfactorily dealt with tend to become more pronounced after the age of forty, and the pressure to resolve our issues seems to intensify in the second half of life. The first half was often so devoted to the business of earning enough to live on, making our way in the world, choosing a partner, perhaps raising a family, that there was little time for working on 'extraneous' issues. When the time comes, however, the repressed material can break out

156

suddenly and destructively. This aspect of our psychology was a key focus of the psychoanalyst, Carl Jung, who laid a very particular and encouraging emphasis on the importance of facing up to and engaging with the difficulties of later life.

Having time to resolve issues

Jung focuses on major aspects of the psyche which are repressed or unconscious during the time an individual is establishing his or her ego-identity ... these aspects must be brought into the light of consciousness in the second part of a person's life.

Dr David Rosen[1] *(see p. 16)*

What Jung and Rosen seem to be saying is that life is about more than survival. Unless we recognise and integrate every aspect of ourselves as we age, we are missing an important part of our experience and therefore our essential uniqueness: our 'psychic wholeness'. If we fail to do it, we will lack some of the happiness which is our birthright, and our contribution to the universe will be incomplete.

I recall very clearly that the transitions in my mid-life were extremely challenging, and remember the depression I faced as a consequence. Looking back I can see that I was liberated to go on a journey, which – though not always comfortable – so far shows no signs of stopping. The earliest and most intense part of this 'transitional life' of mine was negotiated without flower essences, so is less useful for our purposes here. However, I discussed this very point with a woman who came to see me recently.

Case study: Judith
Re-evaluating life

Judith had re-evaluated her life when her partner had left her many years before, 'just as my dad had left when I was seven'. As she reflected at that time, she felt she had been missing something. This discovery led her away from her previous work into a life of healing, of a very demanding kind. Now she came to me **tired** and **sad** – although she was not quite sure why, because in fact she had become almost too successful in what she had been doing. She was moving into the **menopause**, and was once again reflecting on **what was missing from her life**.

As we spoke it became clear to me that she had **not felt wanted** by either of her parents. This feeling had not been fully triggered until her divorce many years later, and it was enough for her to drop her day job and take up a role that involved intense and compassionate caring for others. She worked hard to deploy a very feminine energy, avoiding the traditional masculine model of success that others tried to steer her into. As a result, her mothering needs were being met, but perhaps it was now time for her to prioritise her own needs and desires.

I gave her:

- **Olive** (Bach) for exhaustion
- **Sturt Desert Pea** (Bush) for sadness and grief
- **Splendid Mariposa Lily** (FES) to deal with the 'missing mother' issue
- **Tall Mountain Larkspur** (FES), a remedy for spiritual leadership, to guide her into her next transition

When I next heard from Judith, the tiredness and dragging sense of loss had gone, and she felt distinctly more positive about life.

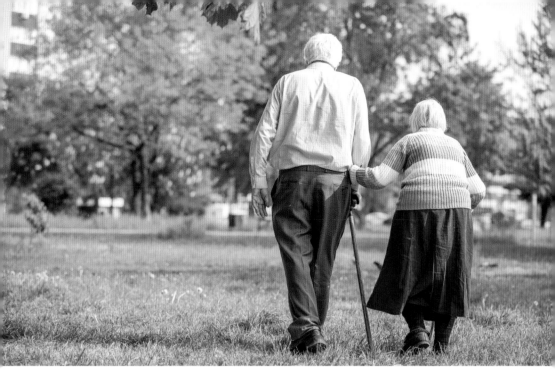

Treatment

If I had my own life's transitions in front of me now, which essences would have helped guide me through them? The answer has to be – all of them! I do not believe that there is a single essence in my large repertory that is not relevant in some way to assisting transition.

Easing transitions

Essences are agents of change. They act as catalysts to our development.

It is true that some essences are more 'transition orientated' than others:

- **Walnut** (Bach) is 'the remedy for those who have decided to take a great step forward in life, to break old conventions, to leave old limits and restrictions and start on a new way'[2]
- **Transition** (Bush)is a helpful combination essence

- 🌸 **Bistort** (Bailey) is 'to provide loving support at times of major change in our lives'
- 🌸 **Conifer Mazegill** (Bailey) is 'for sudden, irrevocable changes in our lives'
- 🌸 **Flame Azalea** (Bailey) 'helps us to regain our vital life force and sense of community after major changes in life'
- 🌸 **Transition** (Bailey) is another composite essence

I could go on, but I hope my point is made. All flower essences promote and facilitate change within us, and help patch us together again following change. This said, there are a large number of remedies that specifically help with the ageing process, and here are a few of them. Turn to page 202 to find out more about selecting and sourcing these essences.

Symptoms	Remedy
Tendency to be needy, demanding, reverting to childish behaviour	**Chicory** (Bach) for respecting the freedom and individuality of others, emotional containment
Dreaminess, awareness moving in and out of the body	**Clematis** (Bach) for awake, focused presence, conscious embodiment and interest in the world
Preoccupation with problems and worries, over-concern with oneself	**Heather** (Bach) for inner tranquillity, positive solitude, emotional self-sufficiency
Chattering mind, obsessive thinking and worrying	**White Chestnut** (Bach) for tranquil disposition, spacious mental state transcending petty thoughts
Feelings of blame or bitterness about life, tendency towards stiffness or hardening situation as in arthritis	**Willow** (Bach) for forgiveness, taking responsibility for your life
Overwhelmed by major life changes	**Bottlebrush** (Bush) for serenity and calm, ability to cope and move on
Poor memory, senility, controlling personality	**Isopogon** (Bush) for recovering memory, relating without manipulating or controlling

Symptoms	Remedy
Overly concerned and worried about ageing	**Peach-flowered Tea Tree** (Bush) for taking responsibility for your health
Feeling that life's purpose has never been attained	**Silver Princess** (Bush) for awareness of your life direction, showing the next step
Loss of identity after retirement	**Tall Yellow Top** (Bush) bringing you home
Fear of death, resistance to letting go of material life	**Angel's Trumpet** (FES) for acknowledgement of ageing process, especially physical deterioration and dying
Confrontation with own mortality at any stage of life, especially mid-life crisis	**Chrysanthemum** (FES) for the ability to distinguish higher spiritual identity from temporal personality
Feeling persecuted or sorry for oneself	**Penstemon** (FES) for courage to face obstacles, impediments and physical handicaps
Over-identification with youthful appearance	**Pretty Face** (FES) for accepting ageing process and allowing inner beauty to radiate
Unable to perceive higher purpose and meaning in life events	**Sage** (FES) for discovering the inner wisdom of life experiences, inner serenity

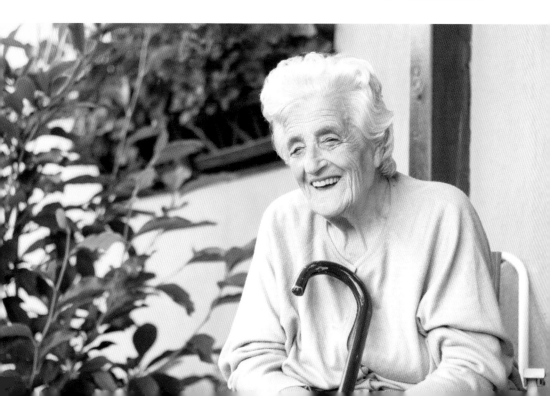

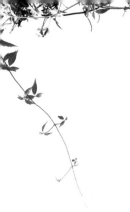

22
Severe Depression and Suicidal Thoughts

Call for help

If you are feeling severely depressed it is important that you speak to a doctor or psychotherapist as well as pursuing flower essences. If you need to speak to someone right now, call the Emergency Services or an organisation like the Samaritans. They will listen and be able to help you.

Samaritans (UK and Ireland) **116 123**
www.samaritans.org
Lifeline (Australia) **13 11 14**
www.lifeline.org.au
National Suicide Prevention Lifeline (USA and Canada) **1-800-273-8255**
www.suicidepreventionlifeline.org

If we seek help so that we can understand the reasons for our depression, we can address them and bring ourselves back into good mental health. From my experience, cases of severe depression often relate to problems in early life. As we have addressed at many points throughout this book, children come into the world expecting love and support from their carers. When carers cannot or do not provide this love or sufficient support, serious difficulties can occur for children. It is important to recognise that children sometimes have unmet needs and concerns in childhood even if their parents are loving and attentive. And parents may themselves be victims of negative programming or abuse from their own parents.

Some childhood difficulties that can lead to depression

- If young children learn that they can't depend upon their carer to be physically there when needed, this fundamental uncertainty creates the deepest unhappiness, becomes internalised, and can cause severe problems later on.
- As we develop, our ideas develop with us, being influenced by those around us, and our soul's blueprint is always there in the background (see p. 25). If our parents contradict our developing views, consistently imposing their own, severe damage may be done.
- Children may suffer a traumatic experience outside the home, without being able to ask for help to process it.
- The disparity between difficult family life and the outward facade of healthy family life can itself become the seed for serious mental illness.

More often than not, problems are absorbed by the family, and repressed by the child in question, who grows through adolescence towards maturity without necessarily displaying signs of disturbance. Indeed, families often wittingly or unwittingly conceal signs of difficulty of this nature from the outside world, until an external event triggers a breakdown of the barriers and mental illness of some description is unleashed.

Depression and creativity

The positive face of depression

I believe that everything in the universe has a purpose. Or, if nothing else, we can live more positive lives by assuming that is so. So what might be the purpose of mental illness? It is often the case that people with difficulty in their lives are the most creative, and that difficulty acts as a stimulus for them to achieve something out of the ordinary. People who have suffered can be more alert, more creatively inspired, more open to and desirous of the new – even to the point of genius.

Often young, sensitive, intelligent and creative people – those 'with most to give' – are particularly vulnerable to severe depression. Sometimes we have to go deep inside ourselves to discover our sense of purpose in a way that does not happen for more fortunate people. If we have no home, we are driven to create one. We may discover and deploy emotions and strategies that we would never have uncovered in a more regular upbringing. And this is what the universe most needs: to roll back the threshold of the known world, going where no one has gone before. Sometimes in the surge of mania, we can think the unthinkable, and break through into another place. It seems to me that this is the purpose underlying serious mental illness.

Divine madness

The Greeks believed that certain people were blessed with 'the divine madness',[1] and that melancholics were rather superior creatures. Not only were the political, artistic and martial heroes of classical Greece melancholics, but their philosophical titans, Plato and Socrates, suffered in this way as well.

Once you have begun your journey of healing, I would recommend that you read Chapter 28 to help you find your creativity.

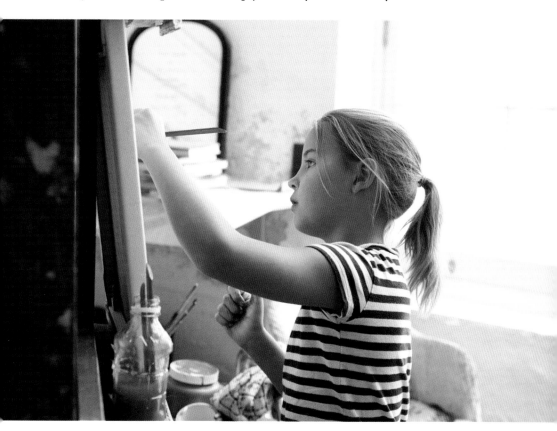

Case study: Brian
Anxiety, suicidal thoughts

Brian had experienced **stomach ache** every weekday for the past two years. His marriage was under threat, he was subject to **intense mood swings**, and he was a worrier who felt 'depressed sometimes'. In the evenings he had **headaches**. At first I gave him Bach's **Agrimony** for his **anxiety**. Eighteen months later his marriage had ended, he had lost his job, his house was on the market, and his rented flat was being sold. While these difficulties were going on around him he had started a training course to become a builder. He had been hoping to develop his own business, but four nights before I saw him he had been discovered trying to commit suicide, and thankfully had been guided towards seeking medical help.

Brian was so close to rising like a phoenix from the ashes of his old life, but he had been unable to make the small push necessary to achieve it. I chose Alaskan **White Fireweed** to support his recovery, which helps with 'deep emotional shock and trauma and allows rejuvenation and renewal to begin'. At his next session he sang the praises of this essence, and was no longer feeling suicidal. He continued with flower essences among other forms of therapy, and I was happy to discover, several years later, that he had established his own thriving local business and had purchased his own flat.

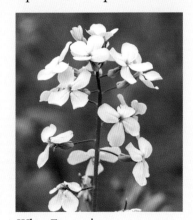

White Fireweed

Treatment

If you are feeling severely depressed or suicidal, try to find the strength to talk to someone. There are lots of trained professionals out there, who will listen to you and support you (see p. 162 for some numbers to call). Flower essences can also help, alongside professional guidance.

How do you feel *now?*

Try to reflect upon your needs without forcing your feelings; if you can, let your intuition come through. Think about how you feel *now*, get to the bottom of that, and select an essence or essences to deal with *today*, then you will be doing a number of helpful things. For example, if you feel **drawn towards suicide**, deal first with finding essences to alleviate the feelings of **desperation**, **hopelessness** and **compulsion**, which accompany that state.

1. You will select the right essence(s) to help clear your present mood.
2. You will build your vital energy.
3. As your energy increases you will enable and strengthen your inner balance, which will gradually help to create a therapeutic 'virtuous circle'.

Light at the end of the tunnel

'In the negative **Cherry Plum** state, people are afraid they may be heading for a breakdown, losing their self-control, or even their minds.'[2] However, enlightenment can come from spiritual pain: when people reach rock bottom, there is often a breakthrough – light at the end of the tunnel – relief that there is nowhere further to fall, and a knowledge that a new stage of development is very nearly within reach.

Significant change, though, can be destabilising and **frightening** – in which case try:

- **Cherry Plum** (Bach) so that growth can transport us to a new place in life.
- **Waratah** (Bush), which has a comparable action. Ian White, the maker says it can 'help weather the dark night of the soul'

Because transition may be too painful to contemplate, you can add:

- **Walnut** (Bach), the **transition** essence
- **Rock Water** (Bach), the antidote to **stuckness** and resistance

Don't worry about choosing the right essences

Flower essences don't conflict with one another, nor with conventional medicine. If an essence isn't needed it will step back and let the others get on with the job without interfering.

Severe depression includes many other disabling states to recognise and deal with, which we will review here too. Look through the following pages to see if any of the symptoms described resonate with you. Turn to page 202 to find out more about selecting and sourcing these essences.

Fear, anxiety

Fear is a common component of severe mental illness, for which I would recommend:

- ❀ **Mimulus** (Bach) for specific fears
- ❀ **Aspen** (Bach) for non-specific fears
- ❀ **Rock Rose** (Bach) for terror
- ❀ **Cyprus Rock Rose** (Bailey) is more powerful and deeper acting than common **Rock Rose**

Symptoms	Remedy
Vague unknown, haunting apprehension	**Aspen** (Bach) for trusting the unknown
Feeling alarmed, intensely scared, horror, dread	**Rock Rose** (Bach) for the courage to face an emergency
Fear of specific things, events, situations	**Mimulus** (Bach) for the courage and confidence to face life's challenges
Terror and all fears	**Cyprus Rock Rose** (Bailey) for creating a protected environment
Fear of losing control	**Dog Rose of the Wild Forces** (Bush) for being calm and centred

Shock

Symptoms	Remedy
Extreme pain or shock in a wide range of situations	**Five Flowers** (**Rescue Remedy**) (Bach) for calming, restoring peace and emotional balance
Shock or trauma, either recent or past	**Star of Bethlehem** (Bach) for soothing and calming, sense of wholeness
Damage to aura, distress	**Fringed Violet** (Bush) for healing the aura damaged by trauma

169

Despair

Symptoms	Remedy
Hopelessness, expectation of suffering	**Gorse** (Bach) for deep and abiding conviction and hope
Extreme anguish, the dark night of the soul	**Sweet Chestnut** (Bach) for spiritual depth, faith derived from encountering adversity
Locked into despair	**Depression and Despair** (Bailey) for seeing the world with a new vision
Dark depression	**Waratah** (Bush) for the courage to keep going
Shock, trauma, despair	**Grape Hyacinth** (Pacific) for stepping back from the situation while harnessing inner resources to meet the challenge, connects to the pineal gland

Loneliness, alienation

Symptoms	Remedy
Separation from place of origin, longing for soul companionship and for meaning in life	**Heather** (Bach) for transforming loneliness into beneficial solitude and self-sufficiency
Holding back from expressing intimate feelings due to fear of rejection	**Pink Monkeyflower** (FES) for the courage to take emotional risks with others

Lack of direction

Symptoms	Remedy
Indecisive, scattered, underachievers	**Wild Oat** (Bach) for showing us how we can serve by finding our true vocation or calling

Symptoms	Remedy
Creative blocks and inhibitions, difficulty expressing feelings	**Creative combination** (Bush) for finding creative solutions in all of life's pursuits
Loss of identity or direction, anger	**Orange Honeysuckle** (Pacific) for inner direction, creative expression

Anger, hatred

Symptoms	Remedy
Inability to open heart to love for others	**Holly** (Bach) for bringing calm and acceptance to the heart
Resentment, bitterness towards anyone close	**Dagger Hakea** (Bush) for forgiveness, open expression of feeling
Repressed anger which needs to be brought to awareness	**Black-Eyed Susan** (FES) for penetrating insight and self-aware behaviour

Controlling, dominating

Symptoms	Remedy
Dominating, tyrant, bully, demands obedience	**Vine** (Bach) for becoming a loving leader and teacher, setting all at liberty
Arrogant, attention seeking, craving status and glamour, dominating and over-riding personality	**Gymea Lily** (Bush) for humility, allowing others to express themselves and contribute, awareness, appreciation and taking notice of others

Resistance

Symptoms	Remedy
Rigid standards for self and others	**Rock Water** (Bach) for flexibility, spontaneity and flowing receptivity

Spiritual confusion

Symptoms	Remedy
Interference with true spiritual connection to Higher Self, spiritually possessed, spiritual confusion	**Angelsword** (Bush) for spiritual discernment, release of negatively held psychic energies, clear spiritual communication
Vague, disconnected, lack of focus, daydreaming	**Red Lily** (Bush) for spirituality and connection to God in a grounded, centred way
Invaded or taken over by other entities often due to harmful occult or meditative techniques	**Mountain Pennyroyal** (FES) for strength and clarity of thought, mental integrity and positivity
Sensitivity to threshold experiences, especially dreaming	**Mugwort** (FES) for the ability to integrate psychic life with ordinary consciousness

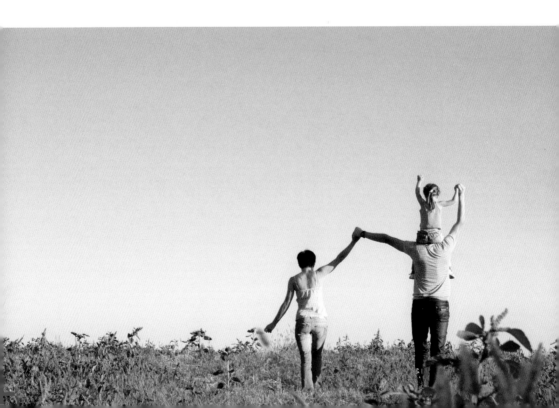

Part Three

The Road to Recovery

Changing for the better

You are the best person to decide whether the essences you've chosen are bringing you any relief, but you should also listen to the comments of those close to you – if they think you're lightening up and seeming to enjoy life again, they're probably right.

If you're used to experiencing significant mood swings, 'improvement' may be hard to define. And if you have been very unwell for a long time, you may be too involved in the process of 'building a home where none existed before' to consider the notion of 'better'. But, in due course, I hope you detect an improvement in your state of mind. By and large, change will signify progress.

In Part Three we will look at difficulties that may arise along our journey of treatment, when we seem to make progress and then stop or, worse still, when we can't seem to make any progress at all.

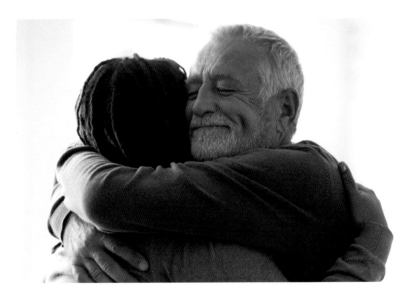

23
Assessing Recovery and Dealing with Setbacks

Nothing's happened yet

Flower essences can take time to work, so please don't lose hope if you feel very little change in the early days.

Sometimes the effects of essences can be felt almost immediately – but in most cases, particularly when we are dealing with complex conditions, perhaps with multiple other medications in place, it can take a while to feel a difference. Essences do not always work directly on the crux of the problem: sometimes they first need to remove some of the peripheral layers we have built up. Only when the preliminary work has been achieved can they move on to the main agenda. At other times we may feel some **uncomfortable effects** as we engage with a process of transition that alters our way of living: for example, breaking with a routine we have developed to compensate for difficulties; sometimes having a cold or fever when we are taking essences can be a sign of forward movement. **If the effects feel too strong,** it can be useful to take a day or two's rest from essences. Simply restart at a lower dose and gradually work back up to the full dose whenever you feel ready. And remember that flower essences are not harmful.

Reviewing your progress

How do I detect signs of recovery?

Somehow you feel right, like your old self. Your spirit has come back, you are more confident. Feelings like this are a sure sign.[1]

Peter Chappell

It is a good idea to prepare yourself to take essences over a period of time. If your illness has developed over several years from multi-layered sources and you have been through difficult times early in life (or you are seeking to help someone else who has) it will take time to resolve your issues. One remedy, however helpful it might prove to be, probably won't be sufficient to rebalance you at once, so it's wise to plan in moments of reflection after a week or so of working with each essence.

If you are **feeling desperate** at any point, try taking some **Rescue Remedy** or **Five Flowers**, which unlike some of the other essences, can be easily obtained from the high street – Boots, Holland & Barrett, and a host of health-food stores (in the UK). While you are taking this, you can give yourself time to reflect upon your choice of essence or essences.

After considering your next selection, do carry on taking the first bottle unless your intuition tells you otherwise. If you have chosen multiple remedies you can put a few drops from the stock bottles into a single dosage bottle. Stock bottles (10, 20 or 30 ml) can be obtained from a chemist and prepared by adding three quarters spring water and one quarter brandy or alcohol before putting in the drops from your chosen essences.

It is a good idea to make a diary note of when you should review your progress and choose further essences. I would suggest a review period between remedies of about three weeks, but this interval is not crucial.

Focus on your feelings when choosing essences; make notes if it helps; trust your intuition when in doubt. If you find you are habitually caught between two alternatives, Bach's **Scleranthus** remedy will help resolve the matter. As time goes by remember that transition and creativity essences are always valuable.

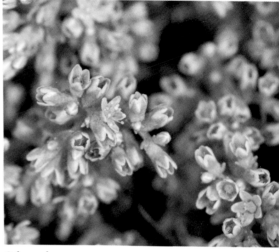

Scleranthus

Later in the essence-taking process, assuming that you're making progress and your energy and trust are noticeably improving, it becomes more and more important to stop yourself from **slipping back into depression**. Try:

- **Royal Highness** (Perelandra) which 'relates to the full stabilisation one must experience when an evolutionary step or movement has been created'[2]
- **Graceful Passages** (Star of California) can also help to stabilise a period of transition and development
- **Walnut** (Bach) for transition

Tackling resistance

It is a sensible human practice to build up a set of defences to protect our developing ego. Whatever difficulties we may have sustained in getting here, the fact is we *have* got here. We're alive, whole, and doing most of the things that other humans are doing – even if we are not as happy about it as we would like to be. So we reason – usually unconsciously – that we don't need to change. 'I'll hang onto the persona that has served me through bad days and worse'. Sure, we don't want to be depressed, but in our experience change can be even worse.

However, flower essences are all about change. That's what they do. They change you so that you can find within you the very best of yourself. If nothing seems to be happening, you have probably not chosen an appropriate essence for your current state of mind, or you have a useful one but you are resisting its effect. This resistance is nothing new. Freud identified it as a barrier to progress in psychoanalysis more than a century ago, as has every psychotherapist since. We are all susceptible to it.

And, appropriately enough, there's an essence to counteract it:

Rock Water (Bach)

Brings us flexibility, spontaneity and flowing receptivity. It gets around resistance, 'softens the soul's disposition and introduces the individual to a realm beyond the hardness of the physical body and the material world'.[3] Because it clears the way for work to be done, it is often used by therapists as the very first in a series of flower remedies.

Addressing fear

Fear is another emotion that can debilitate us and substantially reduce our vital energy, and it is present in every branch of depression or related condition. Harbouring more than our fair share of fear can compromise the healing process.

There are many remedies that deal with fear, but my favourites are:

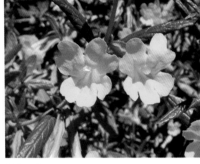

Mimulus

- **Mimulus** (Bach) which deals with the fear of specific things
- **Cyprus Rock Rose** (Bailey) which helps reduce extreme fear and terror; indeed Bailey claimed it was more powerful than…
- **Rock Rose** (Bach) which also has its place
- **Dog Rose** (*bauera rubioides,* Bush) for dealing with fear (not to be confused with *rosa canina*, the English Dog Rose). Helps us towards confidence, belief in self, courage and love of life:

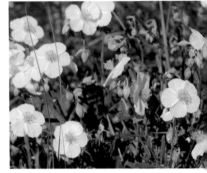

Rock Rose

> being fearful has the effect of blocking and suppressing the life force, the vital energy. Fear also stops love coming in, and it is love that will help to dissipate fear.[4]

Hawkweed (Bailey)

Can be helpful for treating an existential kind of rootless fear: 'There may be a feeling of having been lost in a hellish alien world. Those with some religious beliefs could well feel that they have been damned and are now beyond redemption.' **Hawkweed** can help lift us out of this kind of terror, make us feel more at home and be 'reborn' into a more grounded, balanced state – ready to continue our treatment.[5]

Building self-esteem

Fear of failure can also be related to **low self-esteem**, another powerful negative emotion, which depletes life force and needs early attention in a cycle of essences. It is often associated with **substance addiction**: alcoholics find that low self-esteem pulls them back into addiction on a regular basis.

Chapter 10 addresses self-esteem in more detail, and Chapter 4 looks at substance addiction, but in this instance, try:

Larch (Bach)

This is perhaps the best essence to help improve **self-esteem**. It 'builds confidence to overcome the fear of failure, to spring back after a fall'.[6]

Butterbur (Bailey)

For self-esteem and personal power, because people can suddenly find themselves blocked as they grow: 'This usually happens when they get a glimpse of the awesome power that is beginning to open up within themselves. If they have always shied away from power – refusing to accept their rightful place in the world – then they may become very fearful that their power will become destructive as it develops.'[7]

Hawkweed   *Butterbur*

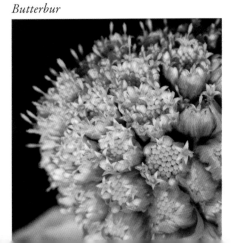

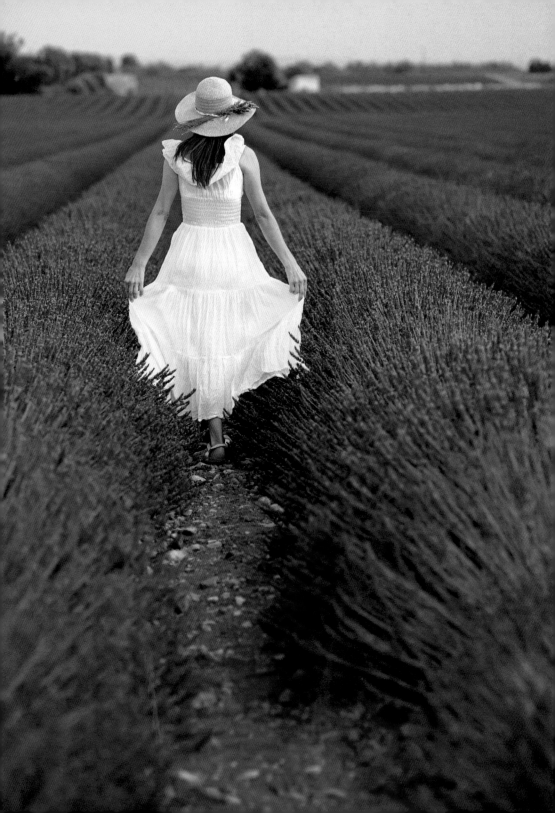

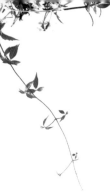

24
Sensitivity to Flower Essences or Alcohol

How many drops should I take?

I get good results by recommending that my clients take seven drops from the dosage bottle I give them, in a little water, first thing in the morning and last thing at night, but for those who are particularly sensitive, seven drops may be too strong a dose and can cause discomfort. People who are particularly drawn to flower essences can be more sensitive than most. If you suspect sensitivity, reduce the dose by half, to three or four drops, as a precaution.

Alcohol-free flower essences

Flower essences are most reliably preserved by using alcohol spirits: brandy, vodka and so on. Typically, essence makers will use around 20–25% alcohol in their stock bottles, which will preserve the essences for a period of several years except in extreme conditions. For young children, alcoholics and recovering alcoholics, or for individuals whose religions restrict or forbid alcohol consumption, there are alternatives.

Wine vinegar or vegetable glycerine made from coconut oil can also be used to preserve essences, and you can contact some producers to request these be used instead of alcohol. In fact, children are more likely to prefer the sweet taste of vegetable glycerine to the taste of alcohol or vinegar. However, these are not such enduring preservatives as spirit alcohol and in hot weather bottles should be kept refrigerated.

Another way of avoiding the alcohol in essences is not to ingest them at all. Simply rub one or two drops on to each wrist (or the sole of each foot, or temple), morning and night, and the essence of the remedy will be conveyed as effectively as if it were swallowed. This works particularly well when treating babies and young children.

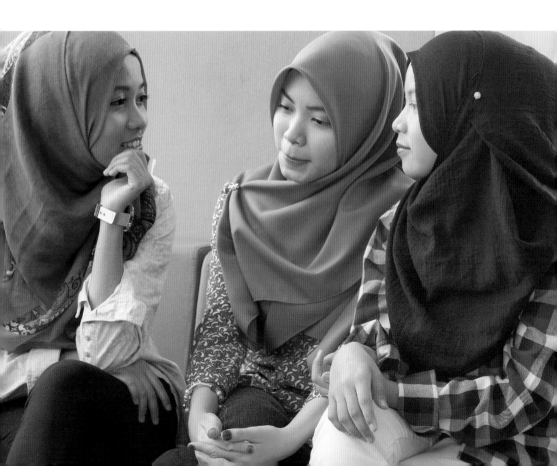

25
Complementary Practices

Counselling

I spent a considerable amount of time studying psychotherapy as I was building my practice, and highly recommend this kind of long-term talk therapy as an accompaniment to taking flower essences. It bears repeating that in dealing with depression, flower essence therapy most resembles psychotherapy. When due time is taken to seek out the cause of our difficulties, the agony and anxiety of depression can be lessened significantly as deep damage is uncovered carefully and the proper connections are made. This is of course great if you can afford more lengthy private therapy – not everybody can.

Tests have shown that cognitive behavioural therapy (CBT) or neurolinguistic programming (NLP) therapy can also achieve results within a few sessions by modifying patients' behaviour, but my concern – and the concern of psychotherapists of all persuasions – is that depression is a problem of depth, and to plumb the depths of the psyche takes time. Without sufficient time, it seems likely that only a surface solution can be found through short courses of counselling or psychotherapy – one that

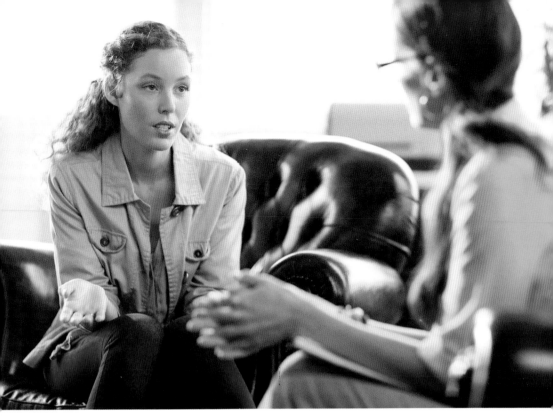

will not stand firm when trouble comes calling again, as it probably will. Flower essence therapy can be beneficial – either to accompany a course of psychotherapy or counselling, or to continue on its own as a relatively affordable, long-term aid to recovery from the roots of depression.

Exercise, meditation and endorphines

The power of nature

I have never felt so carefree as I did then, walking for hours in the day through the thinly populated countryside, which stretches inland from the coast.[1]

W. G. Sebald

There are a number of good things you can do that will help you to alleviate depression and support the mind-, body- and spirit-changing work of flower essences. Generally they fall under the heading of 'healthy living'. A **sensible diet** is important, and so is finding the **right amount of sleep** for you, and the best time to take it. But the most important is to take time in physical exercise that you find enjoyable. Walking in nature – in as green a place as you can manage – is quite simply therapeutic in its own right, for anybody and everybody.

Try walking

> Every day I walk myself into a state of well-being and walk away from every illness; I have walked myself into my best thoughts, and I know of no thought so burdensome that one cannot walk away from it.[2]

Søren Kierkegaard

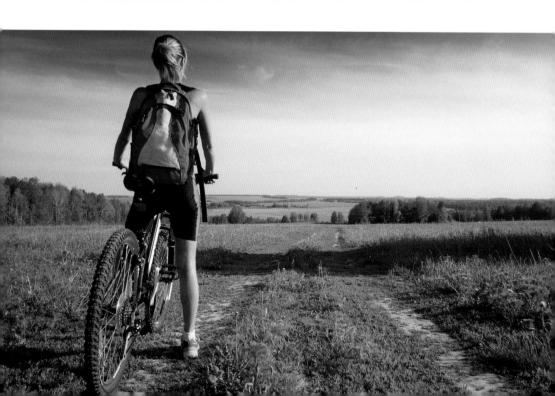

Too many people feel depressed to a point where they cannot take a step outside, and so their depression is maintained and strengthened. But taking exercise and being in nature are great enemies of depression. Riding a bicycle, swimming, even just being by water (particularly moving water) are all highly beneficial too. Ian White (Australian Bush Flowers) advocates dancing and trampolining – because in addition to movement they have a social dimension.[3]

Meditation is an active way of seeking to return to our spiritual origin, which makes it another of the great natural antidepressants.

Blissful meditation

It was even more beautiful than had been described. I was calmly observing everything and yet at the same time I was enveloped in bliss. My consciousness was bliss. The whole Universe was bliss.[4]

William Bloom

William Bloom described his experience of meditation as 'the bliss fields', which can be reached through yoga, practising Buddhism, or through any other form of concentrated meditation. For thirty years, he has been exploring the bliss state and how to bring this kind of consciousness into daily life.

Bliss like this is attained when endorphin biochemicals are most fully stimulated within the body. Frequent joggers experience it; indeed, they find it difficult to give up **running** because of this much-appreciated side-effect. We can all produce **endorphins** – and it's important for those of us who experience depression to remember this. Physical exercise or the deep practice of meditation (or both) can pave a royal road towards such happiness. Difficulties may spring up along the way, but flower essences can quickly and painlessly remove such blockages as they are encountered.

Change your hectic schedule

If your schedule doesn't allow time for recreation then your schedule is simply wrong and needs revision.

If you are working so hard that you cannot take this advice, particularly at a job that doesn't fulfil your creative needs, then it is likely to be supporting and maintaining your depression. A root-and-branch review of how you live your life, and determined action to address any problematic practices and habits you discover, is worthwhile recreation in itself.

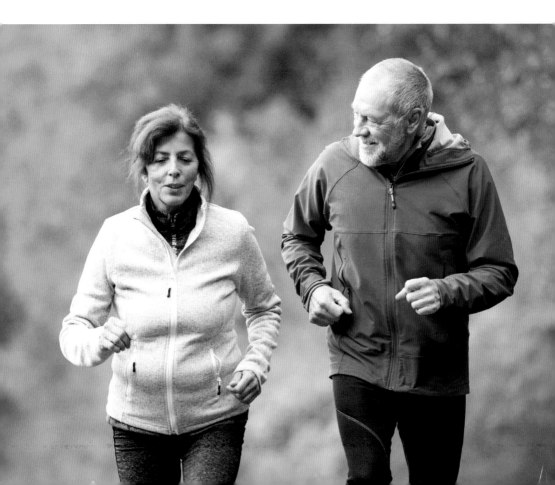

26
Analysing Dreams

Dreams can be very revealing. It is amazing how symbolically relevant they can be to our current concerns, even if they seem totally abstract. There are frequently more ways than one of interpreting them, but our own view of their significance is paramount.

I always enquire about dreams during therapy sessions. Sometimes we may not be conscious in the daytime of the dreams we are having, or we may not be sure that they're relevant, but recurring dreams can reveal things to us about our healing process.

Case study: Irene
Anxiety, recurring nightmares

Irene suffered from **chronic neck, shoulder and chest pains**; at their worst she was unable to stand. She was subject to **panic attacks** and felt that she **repressed her worries**. She told me that her family had moved frequently during her childhood and that she'd found it hard to make friendships. Her parents, particularly her father, had insisted on a high level of performance at school.

Her boyfriend had recently asked her to marry him, but she was feeling indecisive. She suffered from endometriosis and often wavered between wanting to have a baby with him and being ambivalent about children. I gave her:

- **Alder** (AFEP) to help her see life's lessons
- **Childhood combination** (Bailey) which 'helps us to come up to date by gradually dissolving those old patterns'

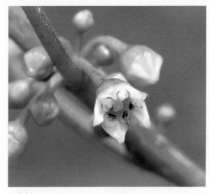

Alder

She came to the second session seeking inner peace, and told me of a disturbing repetitive dream that had occurred over many years. The dream involved a man slowly reversing a huge truck towards her as she lay bound and helpless on the ground.

Knowing this, I was able to treat her with:

- **Mangano Calcite** (AFEP) 'a gentle protective energy that helps us experience absolute safety in the heart'
- **Sphagnum Moss** (AFEP) for those who are 'unable to see the positive side of transformational experience'

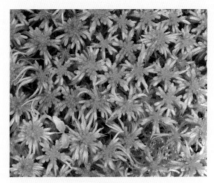

Sphagnum Moss

190

One way of interpreting Irene's dream was that the man in the truck symbolised her father, and that he was forcing her to realise his ambitions rather than her own. Parental pressure or constraint can be an enduring form of 'negative programming' (see Chapter 17) that may distort a person's path in life indefinitely. These last remedies formed an important part of Irene's treatment and we may well not have got to them without her dream.

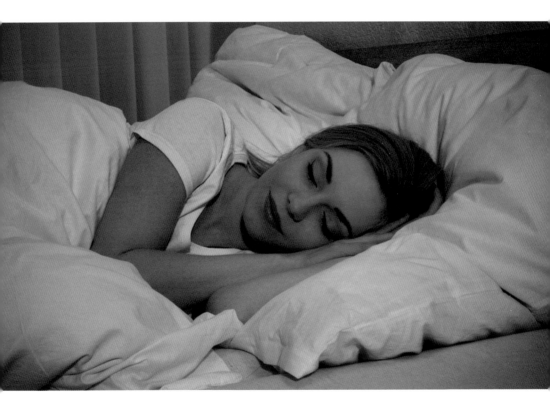

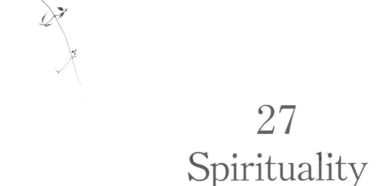

27
Spirituality

Depression and its related states can often be linked to a sense of spiritual longing. In recent years the issue has been officially recognised within the UK health services, in the Royal College of Psychiatrists (where there is a Spirituality Special Interest Group), the National Institute for Mental Health in England, the Mental Health Foundation and in the nursing profession, where publications and research on spirituality have flourished.[1]

Why is spiritual life so closely connected with mental illness? First, I think it is useful to believe (as I do) that we come from a place of spirit where love is the only currency, and the only language that we understand. Our task here in this world is to learn about our material world and to work out our destiny within it. When we are young, our boundaries are weak, so we can easily absorb all the new stuff provided by our family, carers and school. But when very challenging things happen in our lives, perhaps over a long period of time – things that seem to contradict the very idea of love – our boundaries are weakened again and we become open to other influences that seem to provide the guidance we crave. Sometimes these can be harmful (remember Arnild Lauveng's 'Captain', see p. 151) and sometimes Spirit reveals itself very directly in a helpful, loving, personal and useful way, to fill the gap that opened during those challenging times, but perhaps in a way that is not recognised by those around us.

Turning to our beliefs

The cultural context in which mental illness occurs is important, and understanding and integrating our personal spiritual view with our own mental difficulties can be helpful.[2]

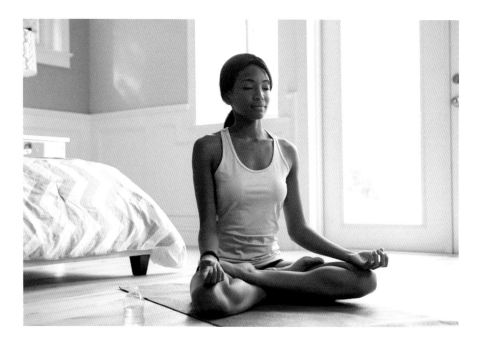

Karma

The notion of karma was included in the early history of the Christian church before being ruled out early in the first millennium, so nowadays much of the western world tends to think of karma as a strictly eastern concept. In any case, many belief systems still incorporate the idea that we arrive in the world with an inherited spiritual task and the soul has continuity through lifetimes. In each of our lifetimes we accrue moral consequences that are not necessarily discharged before our death. If this does happen, we are left with a kind of moral deficit on our death, and a negative burden of karma which carries over to our next lifetime. So we can enter this world with spiritual baggage, and parents have their roles to play in helping to resolve their baby's karma.

Finding fulfilment

While our parents may meet our needs for a while, we soon realise that the only way in which we can truly find the support we crave, and perhaps feel we have lost, is by looking within and by striving to discover our own uniquely satisfying contribution to this amazing world. Only then will we experience true security, and feel that we have come home.

28
The Power of Creativity

I intended at first, at this point in the book, to describe some of the essences that can help us find joy. Surely joy is the antithesis of depression? But thinking about it further I felt this was a false premise. In depression, anxiety and despair we are stuck – held away from our true goal of finding a satisfactory purpose in life. We all have a unique role, and when we are not fulfilling it we can become dissatisfied, fearful and unloving.

Dr Bach was very clear on this. As a young doctor he fell ill and was given a few short weeks to live. In deciding to use his time to pursue his own joy and highest calling he forgot his death sentence, threw off his illness and lived many more years.

Creativity is a path to good health

Dr Bach was completely convinced that finding work or service that is our own calling – our very own creativity, perhaps uniquely so – is the true path to good health.

> We each have a Divine mission in this world, and our souls use our minds and bodies as instruments to do this work, so that when all three are working in unison the

result is perfect health and perfect happiness. A Divine mission means no sacrifice, no retiring from the world, no rejecting of the joys of beauty and nature; on the contrary, it means a fuller and greater enjoyment of all things; it means doing the work we love to do with all our heart and soul, whether it be housekeeping, farming, painting, acting, or serving our fellow-men in shops or houses. And this work, whatever it may be, if we love it above all else, is the definite command of our soul, the work we have to do in this world, and in which alone we can be our true selves.[1]

Dr Bach

When we are doing work we love, it is clear to others as well as ourselves. A friend told me that he had once become enamoured with a particular New York diner. The atmosphere was glowing and the food superb. He complimented the manager and was introduced to the chef, a Sicilian with a strong Bronx accent, who told him, 'There's nothing comes out of that kitchen that isn't cooked with love.' When my friend returned to the diner some months later, the golden glow was gone. He sampled the food but it tasted ordinary. He enquired about the chef he had met before and was told that he had left a few weeks earlier. We can only hope the chef left to start his own restaurant!

Creative people have the ability to tap into the depths of human consciousness and live 'with one foot in the future', foreshadowing scientific advancements before they are realised.[2] By this criterion, of course, Edward Bach might properly be regarded as an artist as much as a doctor. We have seen him being driven in his search for true healing. Only now, some eighty years after his death, is his work being more clearly appreciated as antibiotics and other medicines increasingly fail us and hospitals sometimes spawn diseases themselves.

Imagination is a gift given to us by the universe to encourage us to change and develop our world as we roll back the limits of our knowledge. Our feelings are intentional – they are a language by which we can construct and build our world by reaching out and communicating with the significant people within it.[3]

Essences for creativity

So the final answer in our quest to let go of mental illness is to discover or reconnect with our creativity. Once again, we are blessed with essences that directly lead us there.

Dr Bach's specific remedy for creativity is the seemingly simple:

Wild Oat

> The error in the **Wild Oat** state is one of excessive self-willedness and self-centredness of the personality, in blind eagerness in looking for goals and decisions in the outside world, instead of realising that it merely needs to follow the inner guidance of its Higher Self to discover that the final decision, long since made, lies within itself.[4]

When we are in the **Wild Oat** state, we need to learn to go for depth rather than breadth. Life will not get more boring, as we worry it might, but on the contrary, it will offer us new experiences beyond our dreams. **Wild Oat** also acts as a catalyst to tell us which other essences might help us with our creativity, and Pacific Essences give us two remedies for just that:

Wild Oat

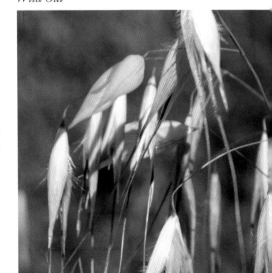

- ❀ **Hooker's Onion** (Pacific) 'for feeling light-hearted and refreshed; nurtures creativity'
- ❀ **Orange Honeysuckle** (Pacific). This essence is important not just for physical procreation, 'but also the direction and expression of that energy into other creative channels'
- ❀ **Zinnia** (FES). The Flower Essence Society has many essences to support and uncover our creativity. One that has come up a great deal in my own work over the years is **Zinnia**, for helping us connect with our inner child:

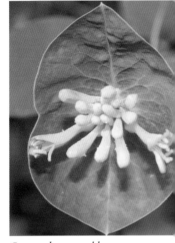

Orange honeysuckle

> Every child is born with the innate capacity to laugh and play, to enter into life with the full exuberance of the winged soul. The adult ego all too often suppresses this part of the Self ... Zinnia flower essence brings the soul quality of humour to one's humanness, teaching that the soul who is in 'good spirits' is truly on a balanced spiritual path.[5]

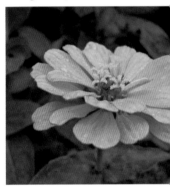

Zinnia

My hope is that if your healing progress has stalled, some of these ideas will give you an opportunity to review your approach in a creative way, and get back onto a more productive and nourishing path.

29
Conclusion

I believe that depression has a purpose. My studies, thinking and intuition suggest to me that the universe itself is a purposeful project. Concepts such as creativity, connectedness, evolutionary development – especially where human consciousness is concerned – all appear to have a part in this complex plan. The vital elements for living a fulfilling life, after basic requirements such as food and shelter, are simple: goodness, gratitude, light, love and play.

Many people believe, as I do, that God is also part of this project, but God is not essential: if you need God then God is there for you; if you don't, you can fall back upon the universe itself for support, restoring our creative energy by getting out into nature in that activity significantly called 're-creation'. For many intents and purposes, God and the universe are the same thing. They grow, they create, they develop and they communicate. The universe connects and communicates with us, making its purposes known by infusing us with and guiding us by spirit.

Mankind itself is one of the universe's highest creations. So, then, it is not unreasonable to infer that we each have a unique purpose, and we are all part of the universe's purpose. Our elevated status brings with it responsibilities, which as a race we don't seem to be discharging as well as we might, but this realisation is itself a spur to do better. There seems no reason why we should not do our level best to meet that responsibility – to collaborate with the universe – to move things forward in the best, most interesting and beneficial way, using all the talent at our disposal. The problem many of us face, however, is that we have to discover our unique contribution to the project for ourselves, 'with a little help from our friends'.

In this highly developed world, in which so many of life's necessities are provided for us, perhaps depression arises to give us a very particular stimulus to discover something special that we can bring to the world. The task of overcoming childhood trauma, or loss, or negative programming is a means to reach this same goal, rather than being the sole goal in itself.

Find your purpose in life

> I believe that the universe introduces us to our proper work in life by giving us a feeling of joy when we are doing it right and misery when we aren't. One of the forms that misery takes we experience as depression. That's the downside. On the upside, we can elect to embrace the project by discovering, deploying and developing our talents, by embracing our creativity for all we are worth.

In his important book, *On Becoming a Person*, psychotherapist Carl Rogers talks of his clients gradually moving in treatment towards what he terms the 'good life'. They become more open to experience, less bound by what has constrained them in the past. Rogers talks of them incorporating the quality of motion, flow and 'changingness' into their lives. They can deal with each new event afresh, without needing to depend on their past attitudes and evaluations.

Leading the way out of depression

Flower essences help us to align our body, our emotions, our mind and our spirit, in order that together they can reveal and then facilitate our life's purpose and lead the way out of depression.

I am therefore persuaded that the universe needs our creative individuality in order to progress. And that creativity, as mentioned in Chapter 28, does seem to be the opposite of depression. Once we have identified and engaged with this idea, the possibility of backsliding is minimised, and we can establish a platform on which to develop our highest potential. In order to fully experience life, we must break down the barriers we have built, and live each emotion or thought as it comes to us, accepting that this is our complete self. This is the goal that a course of flower essences is striving for and, once it has been achieved, we can say goodbye to depression.

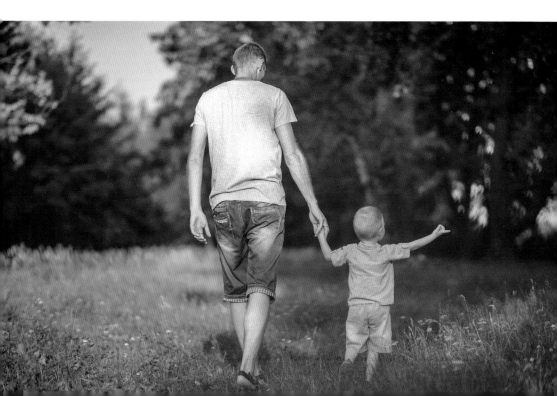

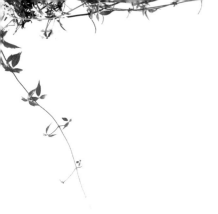

Resources

Selecting your essences

Part Two of this book lists the various essences I believe you may find useful. However, there are thousands more flower essences. My selection in this book is brief, limited by space, and personal. You may find additional methods of selecting remedies helpful, and I list some of them below.

The Pocket Prescriber

Healing*herbs* of Hereford makes and distributes flower essences prepared according to the original recipes of Dr Bach. They are not alone in this, but they do it very well, and they produce a small booklet called a 'pocket prescriber'.

Bach remedies are widely available in chemists and health-food shops or direct from the makers' websites, so it's easy to obtain the essences you have selected after reading the prescriber. My own preference is for taking seven drops of the remedy, morning and night, in a little water, for three to six weeks, although there are no fixed rules as to dosage. You will usually find the maker's own dosage guide on the bottle.

Online selection

Rather than sending off for a booklet you can do something similar online.

Eighty years ago Dr Bach, in little books such as *Heal Thyself* and *The Twelve Healers*, wrote down the mood descriptions that corresponded to each of his 38 remedies. What could be more straightforward than ticking a box against each description that matches your own mood most closely, and then pressing a button that transmits your selections to a specialist supplier who makes up the appropriate bottle for you? This is the service offered by the Bach Calm shop in Carshalton, Surrey and online at: bachfloweressences.co.uk

Selecting essences intuitively

At various places in the book I have laid stress on making use of your own intuition rather than relying on rational analysis alone for essence selection. From the beginning, Dr Bach used exactly that ability 'to understand or know something immediately, without conscious reasoning' to find the flowers he needed. All other essence makers since have followed his lead. Intuition is the best technique for matching unwanted moods or symptoms to the right flower remedy.

Dr Bach's intuition

Dr Bach's friend and biographer, Nora Weeks, describes Bach's own approach:

> Tramping about the country near Westerham, in Kent, he wandered back to the field where he had found the autumn **Gentian** the previous year. Now the ground was carpeted with the blooms of the little wild **Rock Rose**, and he knew it to be the remedy for terror, for he was guided by the same inner knowledge which inspires the musician to write his melodies and the poet his verses.[1]

A friend of mine who is a dentist uses Bach flowers routinely in her work. To select a remedy for her patients she passes her hands over the open box of Bach remedies and 'feels' the essence or essences most suited to them. You can use a similar method: acquire a range of essences and, when you feel unwell or unhappy, 'choose' the essence that feels right to you. That's intuition in action, but it does take practice.

Essence cards

Another intuitive technique is to use essence cards. These are high-quality colour photographs of each individual flower in an essence maker's range. We take the cards with a question in mind, such as 'What essence(s) do I most need at this moment to help raise my spirits?' and scan the cards. The necessary cards should then stand out from the pack, attracting our attention.

Some essence makers who produce photo cards include Australian Bush Flowers, the Bach remedies, Alaskan Essences, Flower Essence Services, Living Tree Orchid Essences and the Pacific Essences – though there may be others out there.

Dowsing

As discussed in Chapter 23, resistance and repression can often hinder our recovery from depression. We need to be able to interrogate our intuition consistently and reliably, and this is where dowsing comes in.

Dowsing is an ancient technique for finding answers to questions where the answer is neither clear nor available through Google! It acts as an 'intuition enhancer'. I find it particularly useful. I use it in my diagnostic work with patients on a routine basis, and have done for years. I hold a pendulum – a weight on the end of a slender chain – lightly in one hand and ask the question, say, 'Will this essence help this person?' and the pendulum swings clockwise if the answer is yes, and to and fro if no. If you are interested in exploring dowsing further then I can thoroughly

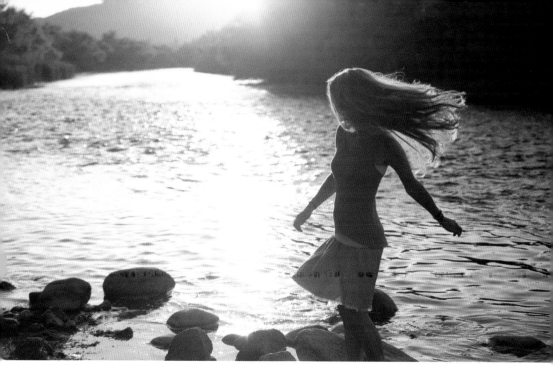

recommend the website of the British Society of Dowsers and their courses for beginners (see Recommended Websites).

Aside from using it to choose essences, I use the pendulum to help diagnose the various physical, emotional, mental and spiritual states of my clients. To ensure I miss out as little as possible, I keep a checklist (or 'protocol', as dowsers sometimes more grandly call it). Here is a simplified version of that checklist:

- Resistance
- Vital energy (ch'i)
- Stress
- Pain
- Underlying negative states such as addiction, fear, low self-esteem, spiritual confusion, etc.
- Past difficulties such as abuse or neglect, addiction etc.
- Depression, other mental disorders and the degree of severity

The essences can help release these difficulties and restore true wellness and vital energy to the individual.

And if you have no idea...

If you have read descriptions online and in this book and still feel at a loss as to where to start, I would recommend that you acquire a set of Paul Strode's Wildflower Essences. Paul is an up-to-date young maker with a well-conceived, small range of essences. He offers a starting box with only eight bottles to choose from and a simple set of descriptions. Study these, think about them and choose the essence or essences that seem to fit your mood most closely. Take the drops as directed for three weeks. Whether or not you feel any benefit, do the same thing again three weeks later. And again in another three weeks.

If buying a box of eight essences is beyond your means go on to the website and read through the descriptions of the essences online, identify one or two that seem most appropriate and order them by post. Pay particular attention to **White Archangel**, **Harmony** and **Sweet Dreams** – they are all handy combinations that have come up in my treatments time and again.

Paul's Wildflowers are the most straightforward 'full spectrum' set of essences that I know. If you get the 'wrong' essence by mistake don't worry; no harm will come to you. They are powerful, but gentle in their action. My eldest granddaughter discovered the box when she was two years old and it immediately became her favourite of all the essence boxes in my chest of drawers. From time to time she would deliberate over my essences, select one or more, and I would be required to put two drops of each directly on her tongue, whereupon she would retire satisfied. I assumed she was using her intuition to choose the essences that were right for her and my dowsing confirmed this. But I could be completely relaxed about it – they do no harm. My eldest granddaughter is flourishing still!

My top ten essences

As an essence therapist I work with more than a thousand essences, so choosing the ten 'best' is no easy matter, but in the context of this book the following list includes the essences that I would find most valuable:

- **Formula Leucantha** (Florais de St Germain) helps diminish the pain of feeling unwanted
- **Red Helmet Orchid** (Bush) deals with all kinds of father issues
- **Rescue Remedy (Five Flowers Formula)** (Bach) helps resolve shock or bad news of whatever description – I always carry it with me
- **Pine** (Bach) for guilt
- **Yorkshire Fog** (Bailey) to help resolve grief
- **Self-Esteem** (Bailey) for self-esteem
- **Confid** (Bush) for self-esteem
- **Holly** (Bach) to help reverse anger, envy and hatred
- **Gorse** (Bach) for hope
- **Harmony** (Wildflower) to help provide a sense of maternal love and support

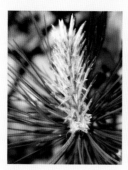
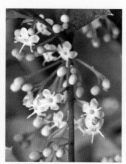
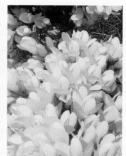

Pine   *Holly*   *Gorse*

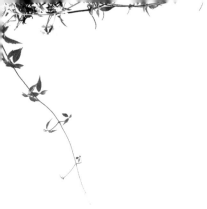

Recommended Websites

Australian Bush Flowers
Ian White's range of essences, as well as a number of useful books
www.ausflowers.com.au

Bach Calm
Website for the Bach shop in Carsholton, which offers the online Remedy Chooser service
www.bachfloweressences.co.uk

Bailey Essences
Website for the late Arthur Bailey's flower essences, company now run by Chris Bailey and Jenny Howarth
www.baileyessences.com

British Association of Flower Essence Producers
Professional association for makers of flower and vibrational essences
www.bafep.com

British Flower & Vibrational Essence Association (BFVEA)
Professional association for flower essence therapists. Some of their members give training in the use of essences
www.bfvea.com

British Society of Dowsers
Professional association for UK dowsers
www.britishdowsers.org

FES, the Flower Essence Services of California
www.fesflowers.com

Florais de St Germain
UK distributor of Florais de St Germain flower essences
landofreiki.co.uk

Flower Essences of Fox Mountain
foxmountain.net

Flower Therapy
My website, for further information on flower essence therapy, how to make an appointment (London) or attend a course.
www.flower-therapy.co.uk

Healing*herbs*
My preferred Bach flower remedy maker, who publish the *Pocket Prescriber* (see p. 202)
www.healingherbs.co.uk

Living Tree Orchid Essences
www.healingorchids.com

Pacific Essences
Sabina Pettitt's Pacific Essences
www.essencesforlife.co.uk (UK distributor)
www.pacificessences.com (international)

Universal Essences
Distributor of flower essences made by AFEP, Bush, FES and Findhorn
www.universalessences.com

Wildflower Essences
Website for Paul Strode's Wildflower Essences – a great starting point
www.wildfloweressences.co.uk

Acknowledgements

I acknowledge with love and gratitude the parts played by so many people in the making of this book.

My first wife Valerie, who knew how people worked, and whose death inspired me to follow flower essences.

My teachers: Julian Barnard of Healing*herbs*, whose book *Bach Flower Remedies: Form and Function* showed me what I should do with my life; Rachel Carter, who gave me my first flower essence course; Ian White of the Australian Bush Flowers, who tirelessly tours the world with his teaching; the late Steve Johnson, who founded the Alaskan Flower Essence Project and helped to keep the flower essence community together; the late Arthur Bailey, who gave me confidence in my dowsing; Sabina Pettitt of Pacific Essences; Patricia Kaminski and Richard Katz of the Flower Essence Society; Daniel Mapel, who makes the Wild Earth Animal essences; Mechtild Scheffer for her wonderful writing on the Bach flowers; Don Dennis, who exposed me to so many fine essence makers (and who is such a fine essence maker himself); Ann Callaghan of Indigo Essences, who makes great remedies for kids and grown ups; and Neide Margonari of Florais de St Germain, who understands so well that the difficulties start in the very beginning.

All the people at the BFVEA, particularly Dawn White, Sara Turner, Jan Stewart, Debbie Sellwood, White Hawk, Lesley Oates, Ronnie Williams, Sheila Hicks Balgobin and Erik Pelham.

All my patients, from whom I have learned so much, be they clients, family or friends.

And to those who helped me directly with this book: David Corr, who read it and commented helpfully on it in its original form – and lent me his own fascinating thesis on depression and flower essences; Kathy Gale of Working Edge, who helped me wrestle with the words for the first draft; and the people at Floris, particularly my editor Lois Wilson-McFarland who, with huge diplomacy, masterminded the version you see before you.

But, above all, my trusty guide in this venture has been Spirit, who was always there in the wings or centre stage, to encourage me when I faltered and nudge me in the right direction. If only I could have let its flawless light through at every turn!

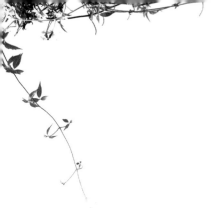

Endnotes

Foreword

1. Barnard, Julian, *Bach Flower Remedies: Form and Function*
2. Bach, Dr Edward, 'Twelve Healers', in Barnard, Julian (ed.), *Collected Writings of Edward Bach*

Chapter 1

1. World Health Organisation: www.who.int/classifications/icd/en/bluebook.pdf
2. Rosen, David, *Transforming Depression: Healing the Soul Through Creativity*
3. James, Oliver, *They F*** You Up: How to Survive Family Life*
4. Miller, Alice, *The Drama of The Gifted Child*

Chapter 2

1. Bach, Dr Edward, *Heal Thyself*
2. Bach, Dr Edward, 'Twelve Healers', in Barnard, Julian (ed.), *Collected Writings of Edward Bach*
3. Kaminski, Patricia, *Flowers that Heal*

4. Jung, C. G., 'The Aims of Psychotherapy' in *The Practice of Psychotherapy: Essays on the Psychology of the Transference and Other Subjects*
5. Bailey, Arthur, *The Handbook of Bailey Flower Essences*
6. Bentov, Itzhak, *Stalking the Wild Pendulum: On the Mechanics of Consciousness*

Chapter 3

1. Wolpert, Lewis, *Malignant Sadness: The Anatomy of Depression*
2. Kaminski, Patricia and Katz, Richard, *Flower Essence Repertory*
3. Barnard, Julian, *Bach Flower Remedies: Form and Function*
4. Scheffer, Mechteld, *Bach Flower Therapy: The Complete Approach*
5. White, Ian, *Australian Bush Flower Essences*

Chapter 4

1. White, Ian, *Australian Bush Flower Essences*

Chapter 5

1. Bailey, Arthur, *The Handbook of Bailey Flower Essences*
2. Kaminski, Patricia and Katz, Richard, *Flower Essence Repertory*

Chapter 7

1. Pettitt, Sabina, *Energy Medicine: Healings from the Kingdom of Nature*

Chapter 9

1. Bowlby, John, *Attachment and Loss, Volume Three: Loss*
2. Scheffer, Mechteld, *Bach Flower Therapy: The Complete Approach*
3. Johnson, Steve S., *The Essence of Healing*
4. As above

Chapter 10

1. Storr, Anthony, *The Art of Psychotherapy*
2. As above
3. Barnard, Julian, *Bach Flower Remedies: Form and Function*
4. As above
5. White, Ian, *Australian Bush Flower Essences*

Chapter 11

1. Kaminski, Patricia and Katz, Richard, *Flower Essence Repertory*

Chapter 13

1. Barnard, Julian, *Bach Flower Remedies: Form and Function*

2. Kaminski, Patricia and Katz, Richard, *Flower Essence Repertory*
3. White, Ian, *Australian Bush Flower Essences*

Chapter 18

1. Freud, Sigmund, 'On Mourning and Melancholia' in Riviere, J. (Ed.), *On the History of the Psycho-Analytic Movement*
2. Kubler-Ross, Elizabeth, *On Death and Dying*
3. Parkes, Colin Murray and Prigerson Holly G., *Bereavement: Studies of Grief in Adult Life*
4. Bowlby, John, *Attachment and Loss, Volume Three: Loss*
5. Parkes, Colin Murray and Prigerson Holly G., *Bereavement: Studies of Grief in Adult Life*
6. Living Tree Orchid Essences: www.healingorchids.com/bloesem-products/

Chapter 19

1. Wilber, Ken, *A Brief History of Everything*
2. Scheffer, Mechteld, *Bach Flower Therapy: The Complete Approach*
3. Bach, Dr Edward, 'Twelve Healers', in Barnard, Julian (ed.), *Collected Writings of Edward Bach*
4. Flower Essences of Fox Mountain: www.foxmountain.net/

Chapter 20

1. Herman, Judith, *Trauma and Recovery*
2. Lauveng, Arnhild, 'When you have lost yourself, there's really not very much left' in Geekie, Jim, *et al.* (Eds.), *Experiencing Psychosis*

213

Chapter 21

1. Rosen, David, *Transforming Depression: Healing the Soul Through Creativity*
2. Barnard, Julian, *Bach Flower Remedies: Form and Function*

Chapter 22

1. Wolpert, Lewis, *Malignant Sadness: The Anatomy of Depression*
2. Scheffer, Mechteld, *Bach Flower Therapy: The Complete Approach*

Chapter 23

1. Chappell, Peter, *Emotional Healing with Homeopathy*
2. Perelandra Center for Nature Research: www.perelandra-ltd.com/Perelandra-Essences-C745.aspx
3. www.healingherbs.co.uk
4. White, Ian, *Australian Bush Flower Essences*
5. Bailey, Arthur, *The Handbook of Bailey Flower Essences*
6. www.healingherbs.co.uk
7. Bailey, Arthur, *The Handbook of Bailey Flower Essences*

Chapter 25

1. Sebald, W. G., *The Rings of Saturn*
2. Kierkegaard, Søren, *Kierkegaard: Letters and Documents*
3. White, Ian, 'Update', The Essence Newsletter, Newsletter of the Australian Bush Flower Essences
4. Bloom, William, *The Endorphin Effect*

Chapter 27

1. Clarke, Isabel, *Psychosis and Spirituality*
2. Geekie, Jim, *et al.* (Eds.), *Experiencing Psychosis*

Chapter 28

1. Bach, Dr Edward, 'Free Thyself', in Barnard, Julian (ed.), *Collected Writings of Edward Bach*
2. May, Rollo, *Love and Will*
3. As above
4. Bach, Dr Edward, in Barnard, Julian (Ed.), *Collected Writings of Edward Bach*
5. Kaminski, Patricia and Richard Katz, *Flower Essence Repertory*

Conclusion

1. Rogers, Carl, *On Becoming a Person: A Therapist's View of Psychotherapy*

Resources

1. Weeks, Nora, *The Medical Discoveries of Edward Bach, Physician*

Bibliography

Bach, Dr Edward, *Heal Thyself*, New York: Random House, 2010

—, 'Twelve Healers', in Barnard, Julian (Ed.), *Collected Writings of Edward Bach*, London: Ashgrove Publishing Ltd, 1994

—, 'Free Thyself', in Barnard, Julian (Ed.), *Collected Writings of Edward Bach*, London: Ashgrove Publishing Ltd, 1994

Bailey, Arthur, *The Handbook of Bailey Flower Essences*, UK: Bailey Flower Essences, 2004

Barnard, Julian, *Bach Flower Remedies: Form and Function*, USA: SteinerBooks, 2004

—, (Ed.), *Collected Writings of Edward Bach*, London: Ashgrove Publishing Ltd, 1994

Bentov, Itzhak, *Stalking the Wild Pendulum: On the Mechanics of Consciousness,* UK: Destiny Books, 1988

Bloom, William, *The Endorphin Effect*, London: Piatkus Books, 2012

Bowlby, John, *Attachment and Loss, Volume Three: Loss*, London: Pimlico, 1998

Chappell, Peter, *Emotional Healing with Homeopathy*, USA: North Atlantic Books, 2003

Clarke, Isabel, *Psychosis and Spirituality* (2nd Ed.), Oxford: Wiley, 2010

Dorahy, M. J., van der Hart, O. and Middleton, W., 'The History of Early Life Trauma and Abuse from the 1850s to the Current Time: How the Past Influences the Present' in Lanius, R., Vermetten, E. and Pain, C. (Eds.), *The Impact of Early Life Trauma on Health and Disease: the Hidden Epidemic*, Cambridge: CUP, 2010

Freud, Sigmund, 'On Mourning and Melancholia' in Riviere, J. (Ed.), *On the History of the Psycho-Analytic Movement*, New York: W. W. Norton, 1967

—, *Introductory Lectures on Psychoanalysis*, London: Penguin, 1991

Geekie, Jim, *et al.* (Eds.), *Experiencing Psychosis*, London: Routledge, 2012

Gilbert, Paul, *Psychotherapy and Counselling for Depression* (3rd Ed.), USA: SAGE Publications, 2007

Herman, Judith, *Trauma and Recovery*, New York: Basic Books, 2015

James, Oliver, *They F*** You Up: How to Survive Family Life*, London: Bloomsbury, 2002

Jung, C. G., 'The Aims of Psychotherapy' in *The Practice of Psychotherapy: Essays on the Psychology of the Transference and Other Subjects*, London: Routledge, 2016

Johnson, Steve S., *The Essence of Healing*, USA: Alaskan Flower Essence Project, 2000

Kaminski, Patricia, *Flowers that Heal*, USA: New Leaf, 1998

Kaminski, Patricia and Richard Katz, *Flower Essence Repertory*, USA: Flower Essence Society, 1995

Kierkegaard, Søren (Tr. Henrik Rosenmeier), *Kierkegaard: Letters and Documents*, Princeton: PUP, 1978

Kubler-Ross, Elizabeth, *On Death and Dying*, New York: Scribner Book Company, 2014

Lanius, Ruth, Vermetten, Eric and Pain, Clare (Eds.), *The Impact of Early Life Trauma on Health and Disease: the Hidden Epidemic*, Cambridge: CUP, 2010

Lauveng, Arnhild, 'When you have lost yourself, there's really not very much left' in Geekie, Jim, *et al.* (Eds.), *Experiencing Psychosis*, London: Routledge, 2012

Marcovitch, Harvey, *Black's Medical Dictionary* (41st Ed.), USA: Scarecrow Press, 2006

Marohn, Stephanie, *The Natural Medicine Guide to Depression*, USA: Hampton Roads Publishing, 2003

May, Rollo, *Love and Will*, New York: W. W. Norton, 2007

Miller, Alice, *The Drama of The Gifted Child*, New York: Basic Books, 1981

Parkes, Colin Murray and Prigerson, Holly G., *Bereavement: Studies of Grief in Adult Life*, (4th Ed.), London: Penguin, 2010

Pettitt, Sabina, *Energy Medicine: Healings from the Kingdom of Nature*, Canada: Pacific Essences, 1999

Plant, Jane and Stephenson, Janet, *Beating Stress, Anxiety & Depression*, London: Piatkus, 2008

Rogers, Carl, *On Becoming a Person: A Therapist's View of Psychotherapy*, London: Constable, 2004

Rosen, David, *Transforming Depression: Healing the Soul Through Creativity*, USA: Nicholas-Hays Inc., 2002

Scheffer, Mechteld, *Bach Flower Therapy: The Complete Approach*, London: Thorsons, 2009

Sebald, W. G., *The Rings of Saturn*, London: Vintage, 2002

Storr, Anthony, *The Art of Psychotherapy* (2nd Ed), New York: Routledge, 1990

Weeks, Nora, *The Medical Discoveries of Edward Bach*, Physician, Saffron Walden: C. W. Daniel Company, 2007 (1940)

White, Ian, *Australian Bush Flower Essences*, UK: Findhorn Press, 1991

—, *Bush Flower Healing*, London: Bantam, 1999

—, 'Update', The Essence Newsletter, Newsletter of the Australian Bush Flower Essences, Bush Biotherapies Pty Ltd, June 2010

Wilber, Ken, *The Atman Project: A Transpersonal View of Human Development*, USA: Quest Books, 1996

—, *A Brief History of Everything*, USA: Shambhala Publications, 2017

Wolpert, Lewis, *Malignant Sadness: The Anatomy of Depression*, London: Faber & Faber, 1999

Zaalberg, Bram, *Flower Essences: A Gift of Nature. Maker's Catalogue*, www.healingorchids.com

Index of Essences

Healing Plants
Herbal Remedies from Traditional to Anthroposophical Medicine

Dr Markus Sommer

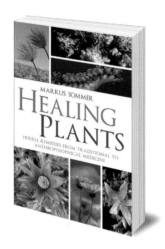

More than just a simple guide to herbal remedies, this book lifts the lid on the powerful secrets of the plant world.

In this illustrated, readable book Dr Markus Sommer vividly describes the properties of over thirty plants, helping the reader to understand their true nature. For example, did you know that St John's Wort is not only good for depression, but also heals wounds? Plantain is good for coughs, but is also effective in treating strokes and multiple sclerosis.

Dr Sommer demonstrates the deep connection between the character of the plant and the nature of the conditions they can cure or alleviate.

florisbooks.co.uk

Bach Flower Remedies
Form and Function

Julian Barnard

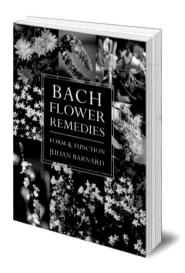

In the 1920s, the physician and homeopath Dr Edward Bach made his great discovery of the healing effects of various flower essences, which resulted in thirty-eight 'flower remedies'. Bach described them as 'bringing courage to the fearful, peace to the anguished, and strength to the weak', but the therapeutic effects of the remedies go beyond emotional states. They are equally effective in the treatment of physical disorders.

Julian Barnard describes how Bach made his discoveries, examines the living qualities of the plants in their context, and looks at how the remedies are actually produced. The result is remarkable. Barnard recounts his observations so that readers can experience for themselves the complex ways in which the remedy plants grow.

florisbooks.co.uk

An Illustrated Guide to Everyday Eurythmy
Discover Balance and Self-Healing through Movement

Barbara Tapfer & Annette Weisskircher

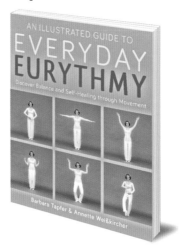

Discover the art of eurythmy with this richly illustrated step-by-step guide.

Eurythmy is a compelling method of bringing balance and harmony to our body, soul and spirit through a series of rhythmic body movements. For the first time, this unique book captures these gestures visually through dynamic photographs, which clearly demonstrate the core movements of eurythmy therapy.

The authors of this original book are experienced eurythmists, who describe and illustrate the core speech-sound exercises: vowel exercises, consonant exercises and soul exercises, which include love, hope and sympathy.

florisbooks.co.uk

Lowering High Blood Pressure
The Three-type Holistic Approach

Dr Thomas Breitkreuz & Annette Bopp

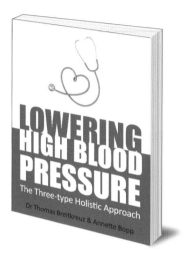

This book offers a tailored and holistic programme for anyone who suffers from high blood pressure, distinguishing between three core types of hypertension: stress type, abdominal type, and chaos type.

The authors of this accessible book, including an experienced physician, want to empower you to discover a new way to treat high blood pressure, outside of conventional treatments. Once you have identified which of the three core types of high blood pressure you have, you can follow the tailor-made therapeutic programmes which care for body and soul, including nutrition, exercise and anthroposophical therapies to suit each type.

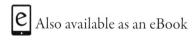 Also available as an eBook

florisbooks.co.uk

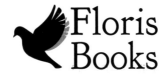

Floris Books

For news on all our **latest books**,
and to receive **exclusive discounts**,
join our mailing list at:

florisbooks.co.uk

Plus subscribers get a FREE book
with every online order!